Let's Be Critical Thinkers

CRITICALLY THINKING ABOUT MASKS, LOCKDOWNS, SOCIAL DISTANCING & VACCINES

Skyhorse Publishing books may be purchased in bulk at special discounts for sales promotion, corporate gifts, fund-raising, or educational purposes. Special editions can also be created to specifications. For details, contact the Special Sales Department, Skyhorse Publishing, 307 West 36th Street, 11th Floor, New York, NY 10018 or info@skyhorsepublishing.com.

Skyhorse® and Skyhorse Publishing® are registered trademarks of Skyhorse Publishing, Inc.®, a Delaware corporation.

Visit our website at www.skyhorsepublishing.com.

10 9 8 7 6 5 4 3 2 1

Manufactured in China, June 2025
This product conforms to CPSIA 2008

Library of Congress Cataloging-in-Publication Data is available on file.

Hardcover ISBN: 978-1-5107-8464-2
Ebook ISBN: 978-1-5107-8465-9

Cover design by Manfred Calderón
Cover illustration by Manfred Calderón

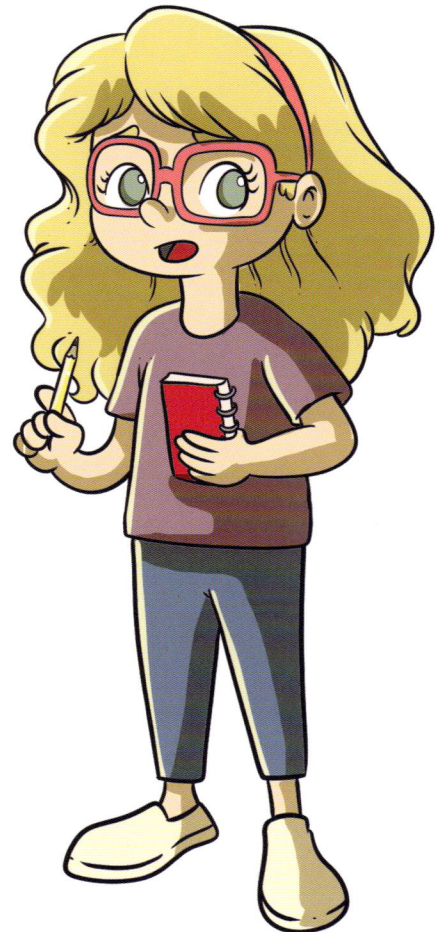

Let's Be Critical Thinkers

CRITICALLY THINKING ABOUT MASKS, LOCKDOWNS, SOCIAL DISTANCING & VACCINES

Written by Dr. Shannon Kroner

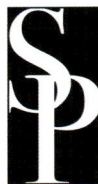

Illustrated by Manfred Calderón

A few things to know before reading *Let's Be Critical Thinkers*:

- All studies mentioned in this book can be found on the reference page.
- This book has some big words that are further explained in the glossary.
- You'll also find some fun, critical thinking activities at the end of this book.
- A special thank you to Dr. Joseph Ladapo, Dr. James Lyons-Weiler, Dr. Jeff Barke, and Dr. Judy Mikovits for their part in this story.
- Most importantly, I hope you enjoy reading my book. I enjoyed writing it.
  ~Dr. Shannon Kroner

Skyhorse Publishing, Inc.

Dedications

To the investigative journalists and influencers who make it their job to search for facts and share the truth, despite the risks of censorship.

To the doctors and scientists who understand that science is never settled and have risked their practices and licenses in pursuit of medical truths.

To our military, first responders, teachers, and nurses who were forced to choose between their careers and their health, and still fought to be heard.

To the parents and kids who embrace free thinking, staying open to new ideas and new perspectives.

To my talented illustrator who turned all my ideas into beautiful illustrations.

To my friends, for their heartfelt encouragement and insightful feedback.

To my husband, whose boundless enthusiasm and support fueled my creative spark throughout the process of creating this book.

To my boys, for their unique insights and smart suggestions, which helped inspire this story and truly capture the pandemic through a child's eyes.

To my mom, for her love, support, and the pride she beams when she shares my books with others.

Thank you.

Wise Words from Critical Thinkers

"Dr. Kroner's, *Let's Be Critical Thinkers* provides our nation's youth with the tools to seek the truth and question the narrative through essential access to complex, empowering ideas and knowledge in an accurate and easy-to-grasp presentation. This book will inspire young minds to think critically and stay curious about the world; for it is through questioning and exploration that we uncover truth and grow wiser. Any parent should be proud of their child who begins to ask questions after reading this book."
—JAMES LYONS-WEILER, PHD, author, CEO, scientist, editor-in-chief of *Science, Public Health Policy, and the Law*, and founder of Popular Rationalism

"My wife, Brianna, and I work hard to teach our kids how to think critically. As parents, it is one of the greatest gifts we can bestow on our children—and perhaps more important than ever because of the Information Age. Dr. Shannon Kroner's book is not only fun to read but also a treasure for the young minds who pursue its pages and for parents who are seeking healthy ways to reinforce the invaluable tool of critical thinking."
—JOSEPH LADAPO, MD, author of *Transcend Fear: A Blueprint for Mindful Leadership in Public Health*, professor at University of Florida College of Medicine, and Surgeon General of Florida

"Dr. Shannon Kroner has done it again with her eye-opening children's book about the insane policies implemented during COVID. Critical thinking is sorely missing in our post-COVID era, and Dr. Kroner points out the obvious past failures and opportunities ahead. Although written for children, even adults will benefit from the information! This book will be proudly displayed in my medical office for both parents and children!"
—JEFFREY I. BARKE, MD, author of *Unavoidably Unsafe: Childhood Vaccines Reconsidered*

"Dr. Shannon Kroner's *Let's Be Critical Thinkers* is a wonderful guide for children to learn how to think for themselves. In today's world, it's important for kids to ask questions, seek the truth, and understand what's happening around them. This book helps young minds grow strong and curious, empowering them to make sense of the world with kindness and clarity."
—JUDY A. MIKOVITS, PHD, biochemistry and molecular biology, *New York Times* bestselling author of *Plague of Corruption*

"As a firefighter who stood up against unfair vaccine mandates, I experienced the deep frustration of losing my freedom—and even my job. Being terminated took away my God-given, constitutional right to earn a living and provide for my family. *Let's Be Critical Thinkers* tells that story through the eyes of a curious child searching for truth. Dr. Kroner powerfully captures what first responders like myself went through by helping kids understand the importance of thinking for themselves and standing up for what's right. Critical thinking needs to be taught again, and this book gets it right."
—JOHN KNOX, firefighter/paramedic, co-founder of Firefighters 4 Freedom, and HHS principal deputy assistant secretary for preparedness and response

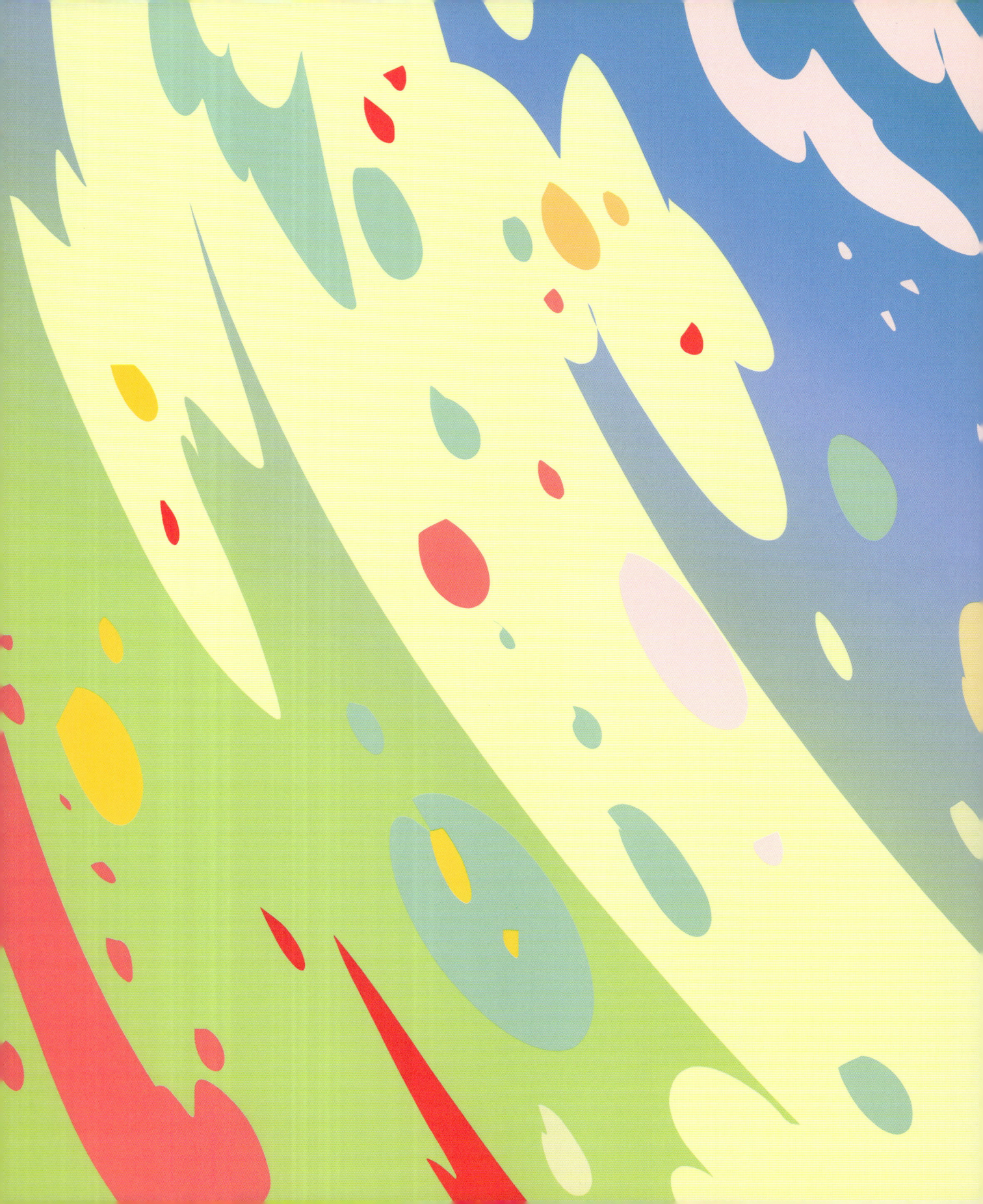

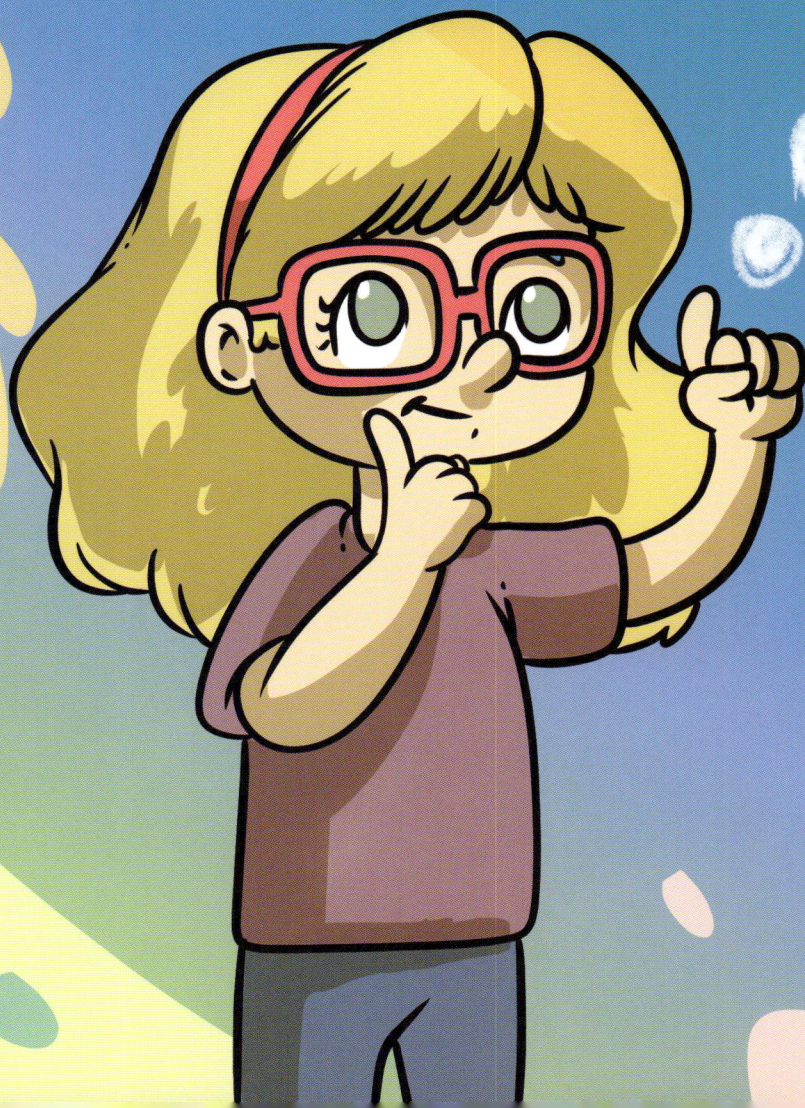

PART ONE:

HOW TO BE A
CRITICAL THINKER

Hello. My name is Darlene Data, and I love doing research.

When I grow up, I want to be an investigative journalist.

Good investigative journalists ask smart questions, look for answers, and are truthful about what they find.

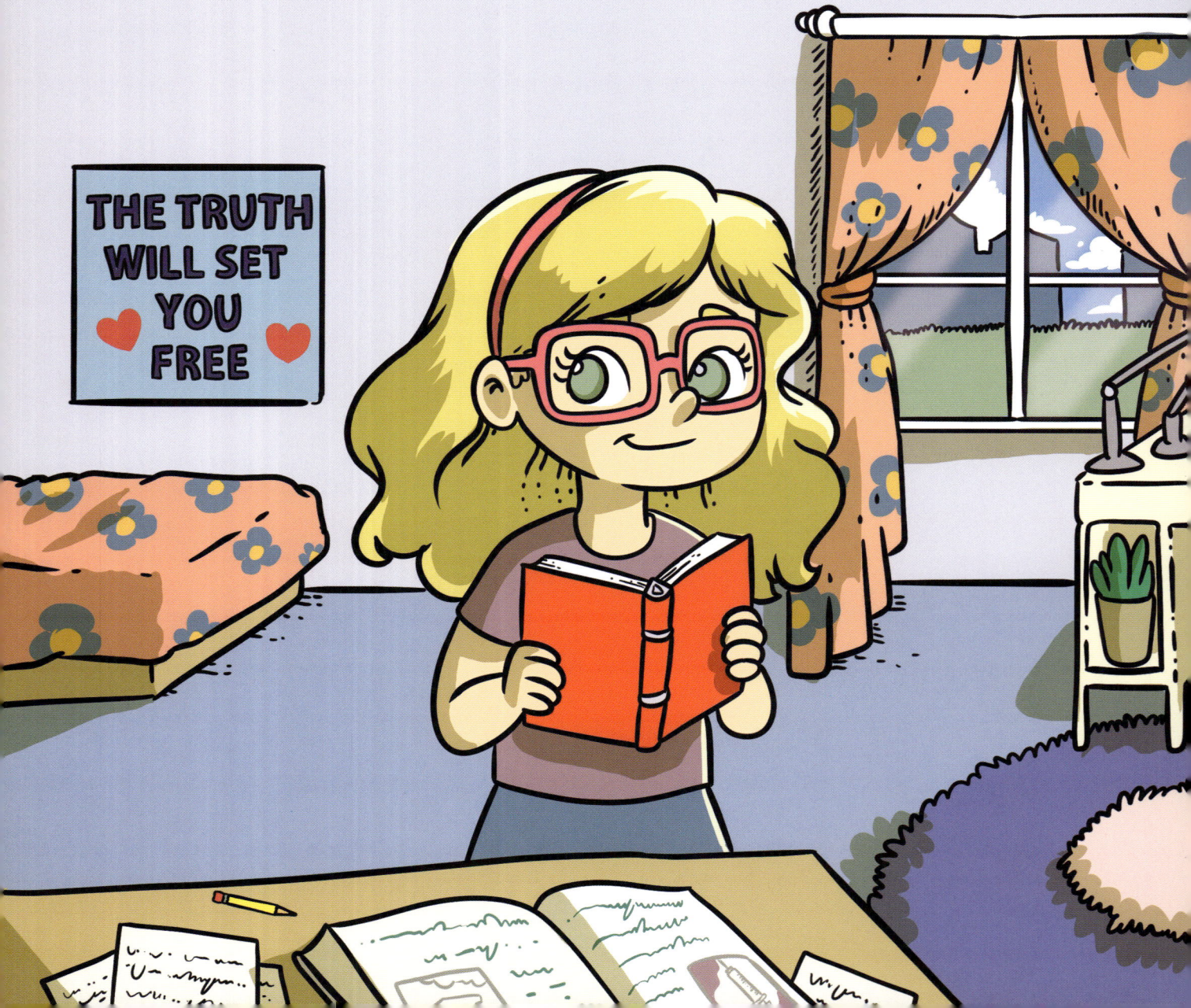

THE TRUTH WILL SET YOU FREE

In the year 2020, the world experienced a global pandemic. While our government looked for ways to manage it, society was given lots of confusing information about masks, lockdowns, social distancing, and vaccines.

Many people were unsure how to respond to the confusion and didn't know what to believe.

So I've decided to investigate the information, and separate the facts from the fiction! I hope you'll join me on this adventure in critical thinking.

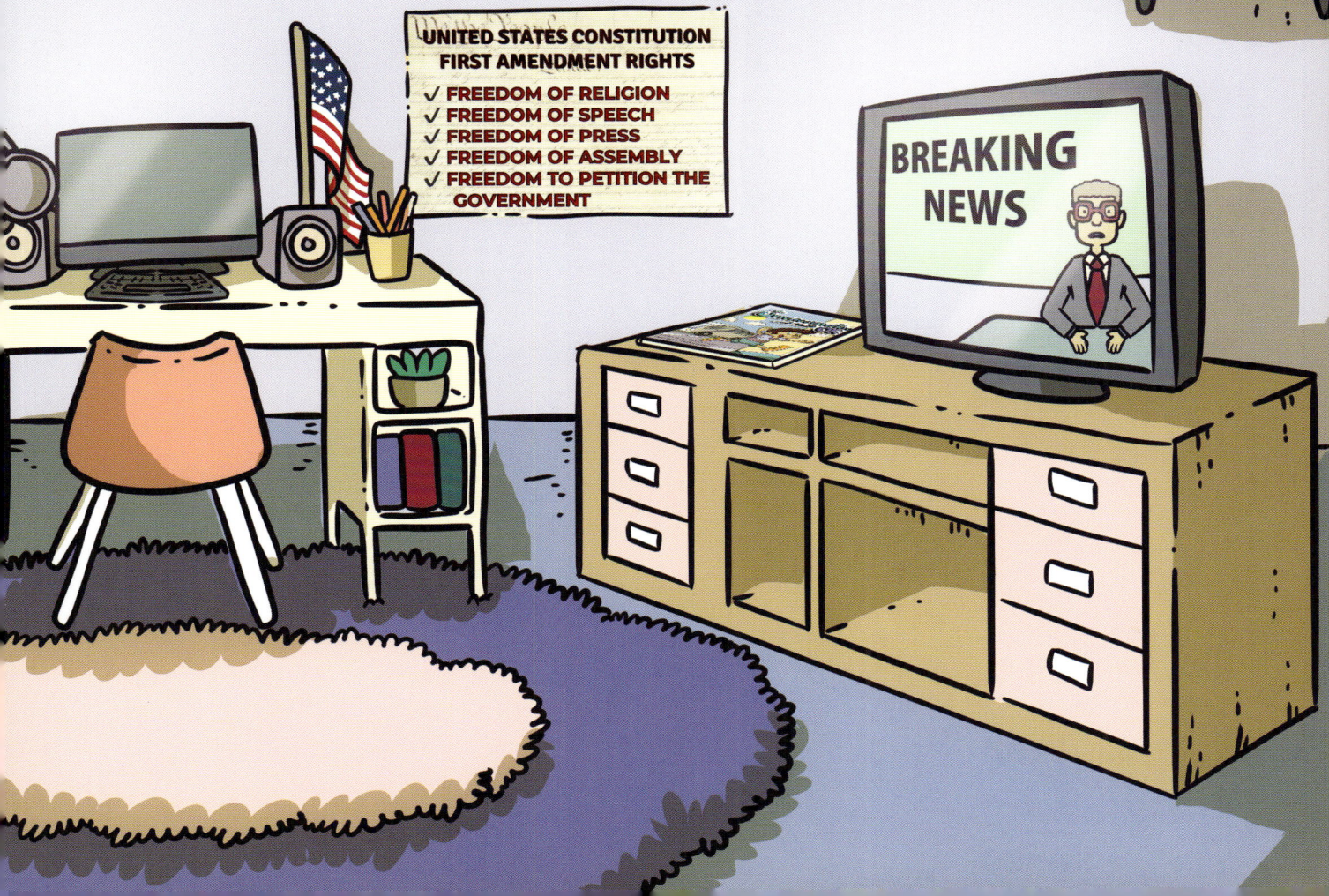

UNITED STATES CONSTITUTION
FIRST AMENDMENT RIGHTS
✓ FREEDOM OF RELIGION
✓ FREEDOM OF SPEECH
✓ FREEDOM OF PRESS
✓ FREEDOM OF ASSEMBLY
✓ FREEDOM TO PETITION THE GOVERNMENT

BREAKING NEWS

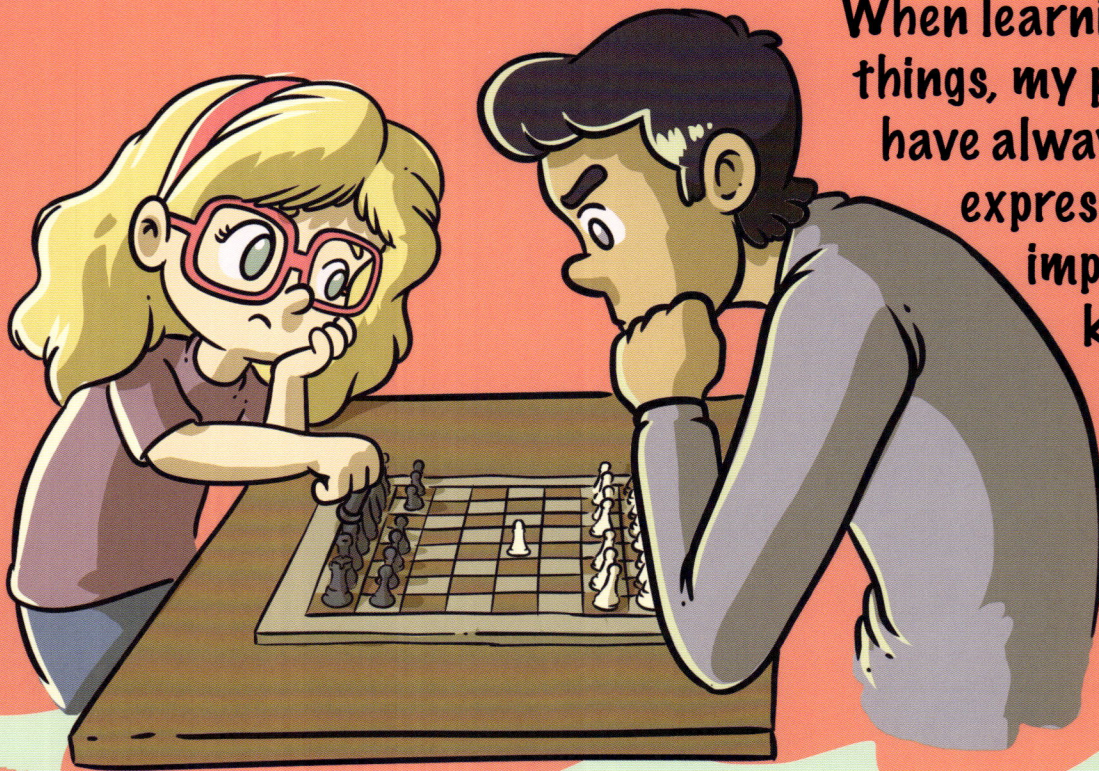

When learning new things, my parents have always expressed the importance of keeping an open and independent mind.

They encourage me to gather information, look at the whole puzzle to see where the pieces fit, and form my own opinions based on what I've put together.

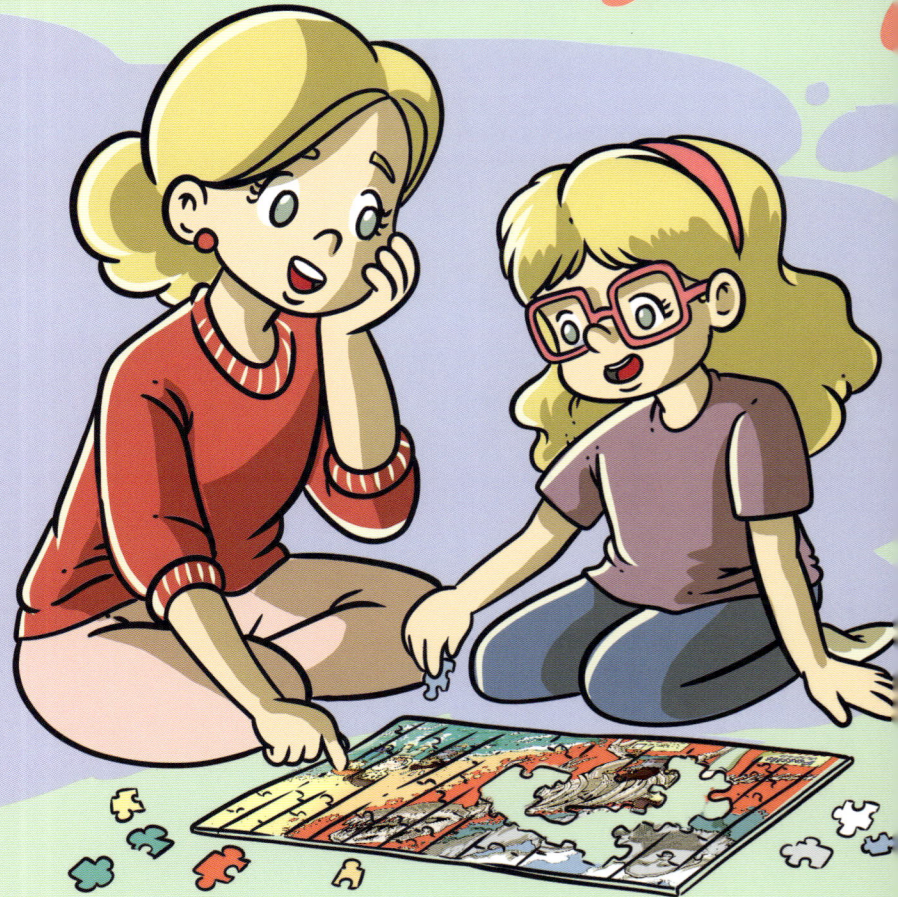

Even though we should be able to trust our government and what the news tells us, I've also been taught that it's important to ask questions.

When examining current events, people should always consider the bigger picture and ask WHY someone is saying or doing something.

This is called critical thinking.

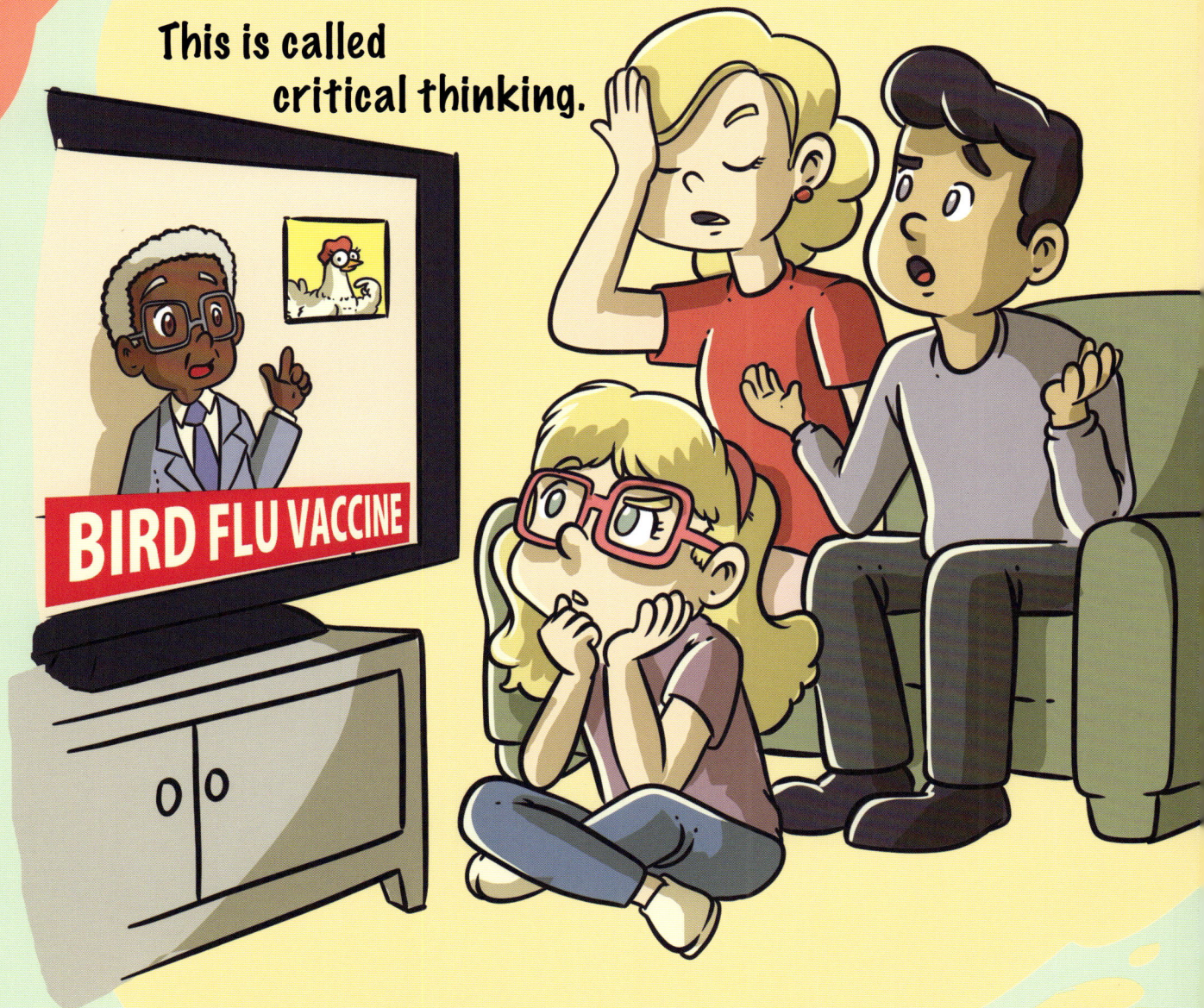

BIRD FLU VACCINE

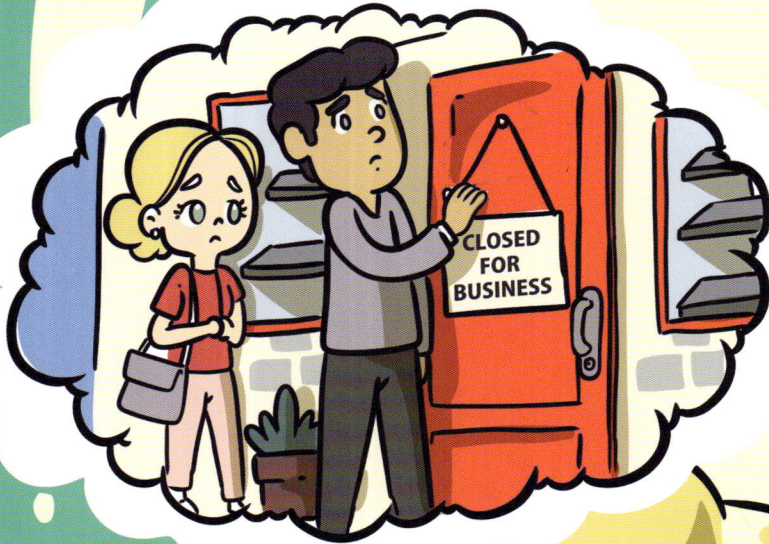

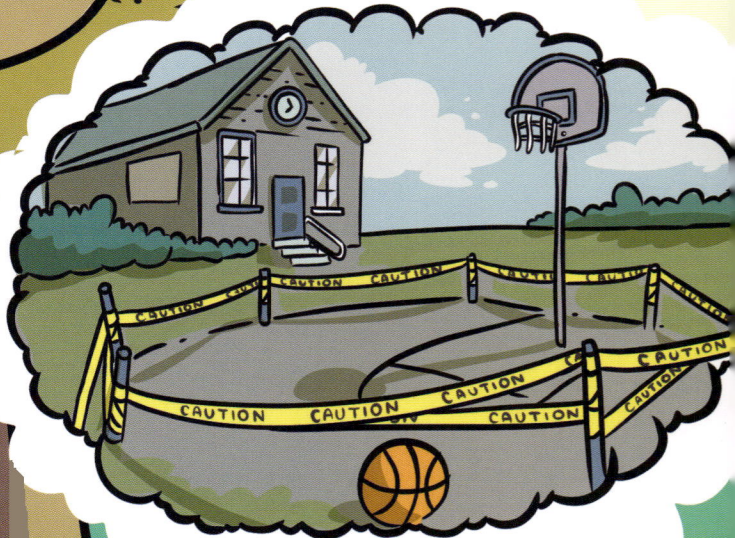

Many people reacted out of fear without using any critical thinking skills or questioning what they were being instructed to do.

Some people wore masks at all times and were scared to breathe fresh air.

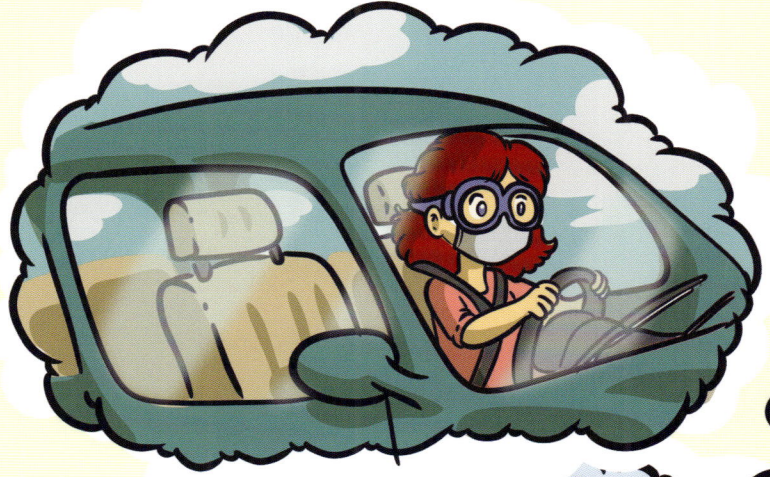

Others made sure to stay six feet away from one another to reduce the spread of germs.

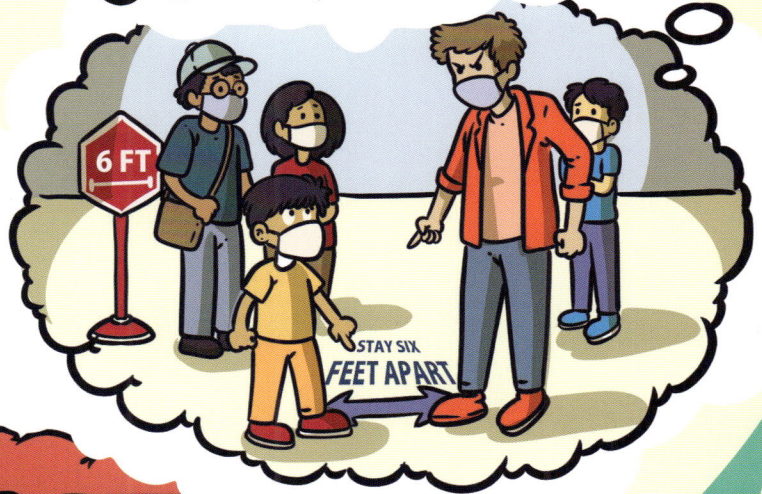

Businesses made up new rules deciding who was and wasn't allowed to enter.

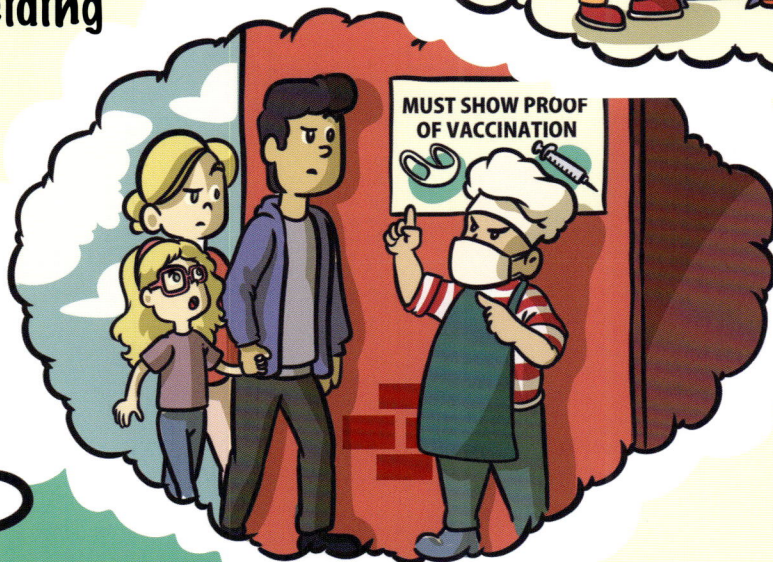

Throughout America, many businesses placed signs on their doors and windows saying, "Must show proof of vaccination" and "Do not enter without a mask."

Suddenly, my family and I weren't allowed into our favorite restaurants or businesses because of our vaccine status!

These rules were intended to help keep people safe, but they were unfair to those who may not have been able to wear a mask or get vaccinated.

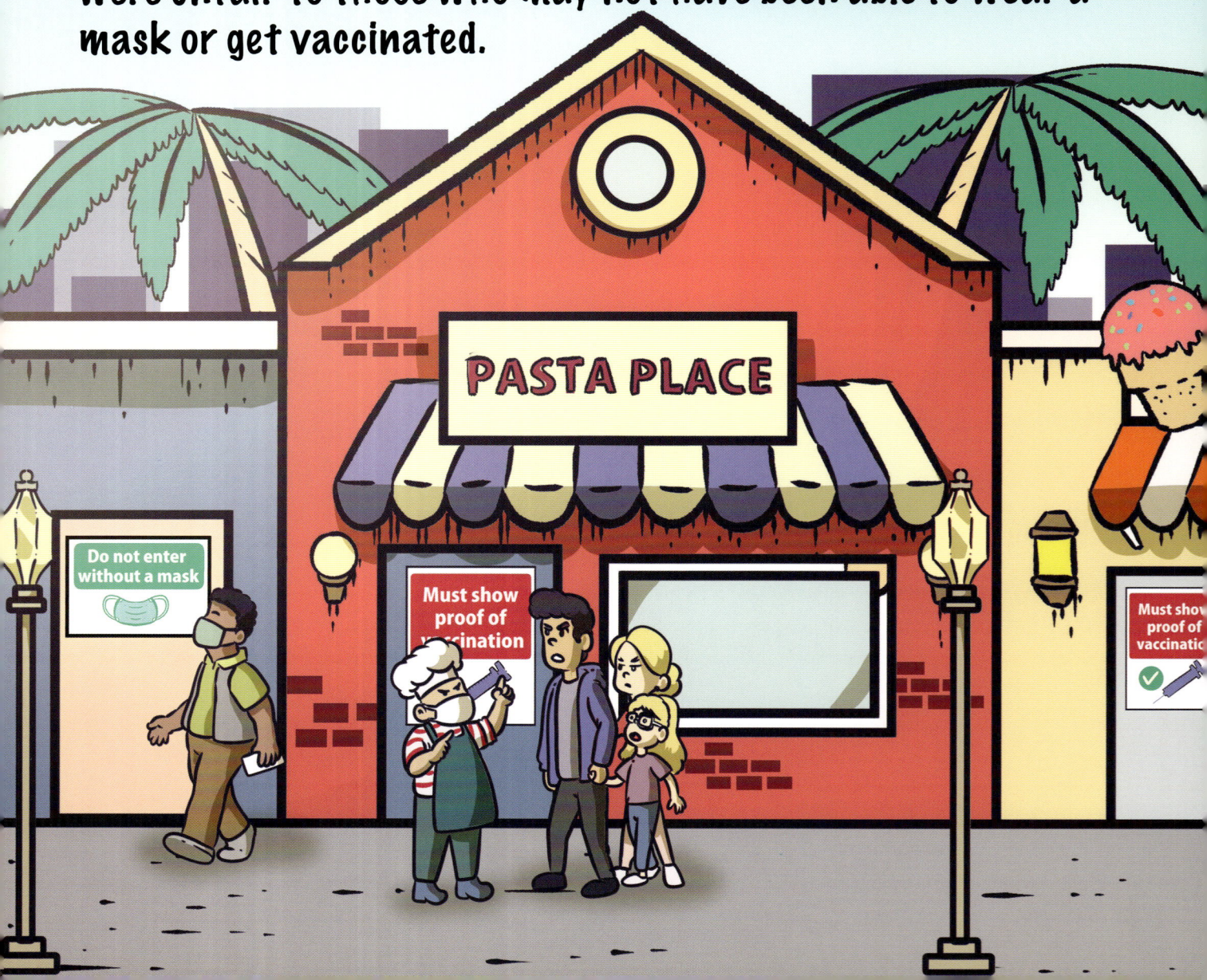

These rules also didn't make much sense.

How did wearing a mask to enter a restaurant prevent people from spreading germs, especially if they were allowed to take off their masks while sipping on a drink or eating food?

And, if vaccinated people were protected by their vaccines, then why did it matter if those around them weren't vaccinated?

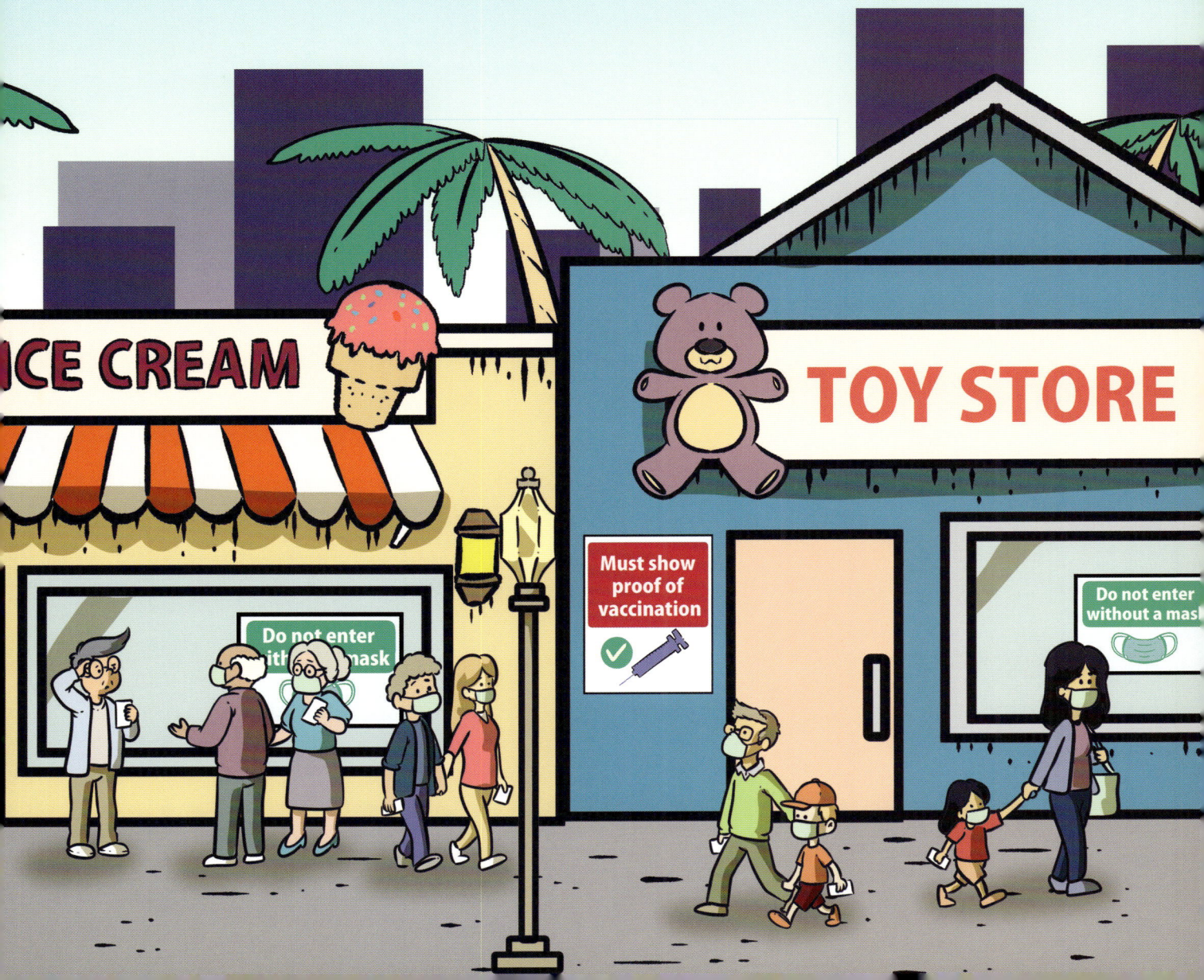

ICE CREAM

TOY STORE

Do not enter without a mask

Must show proof of vaccination

Do not enter without a mask

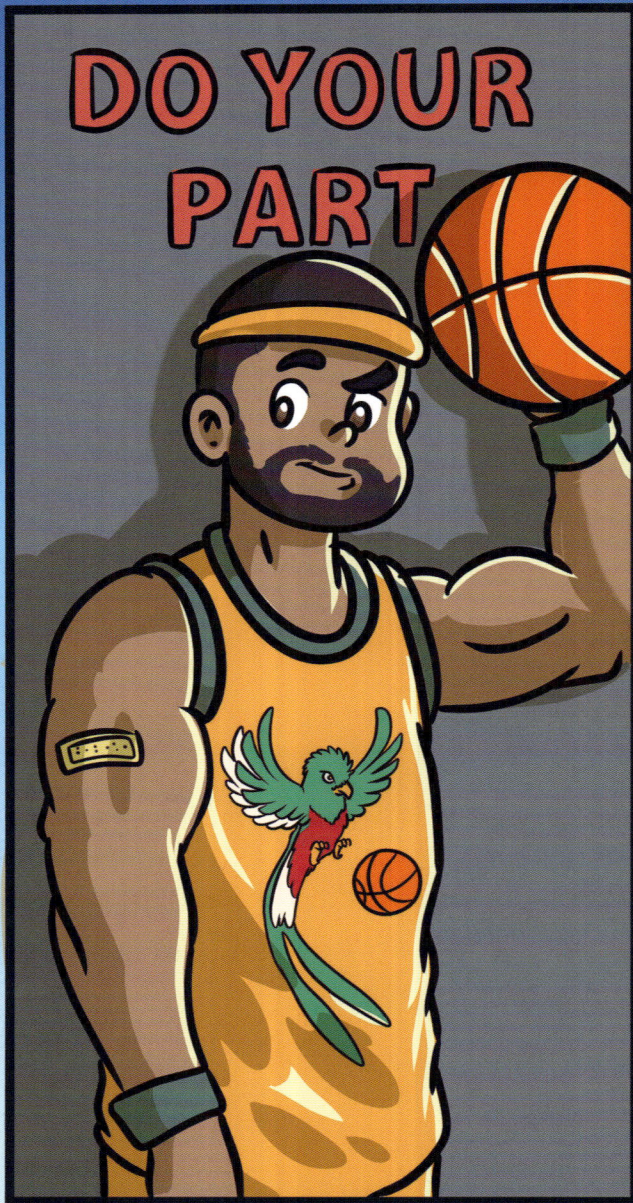

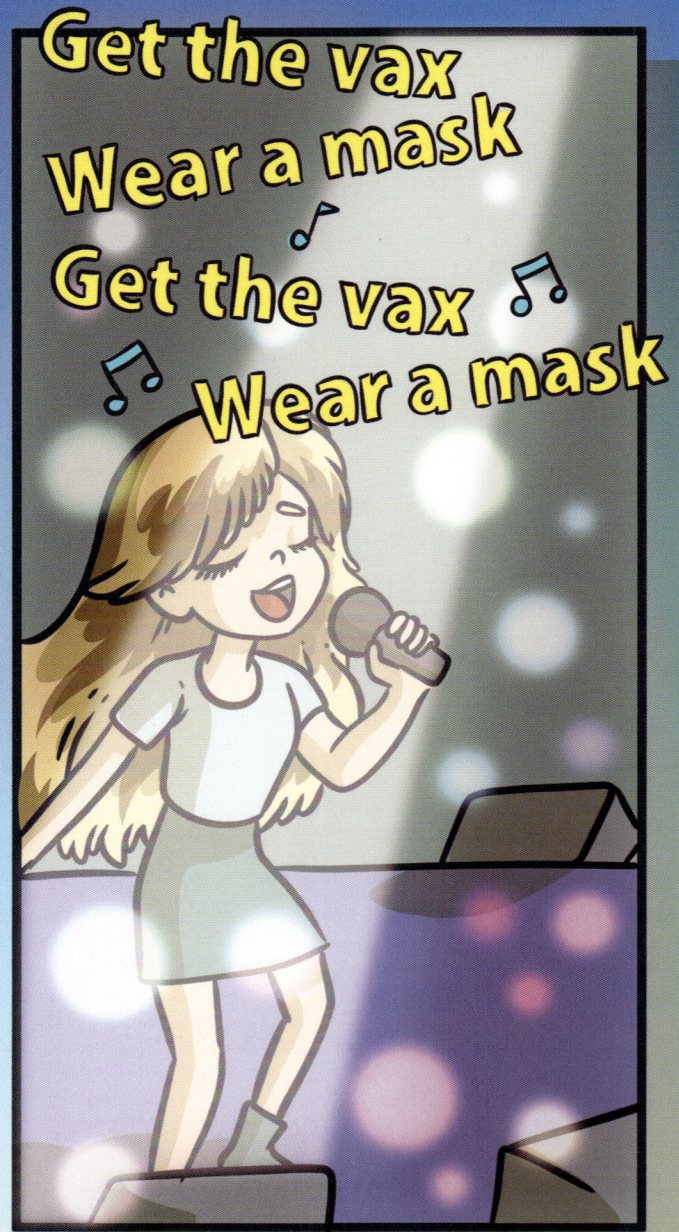

Athletes and celebrities also encouraged the public to get vaccinated and wear a mask everywhere they went.

The news repeatedly told the public how bad things were, and how much worse it may get if they didn't do what they were told.

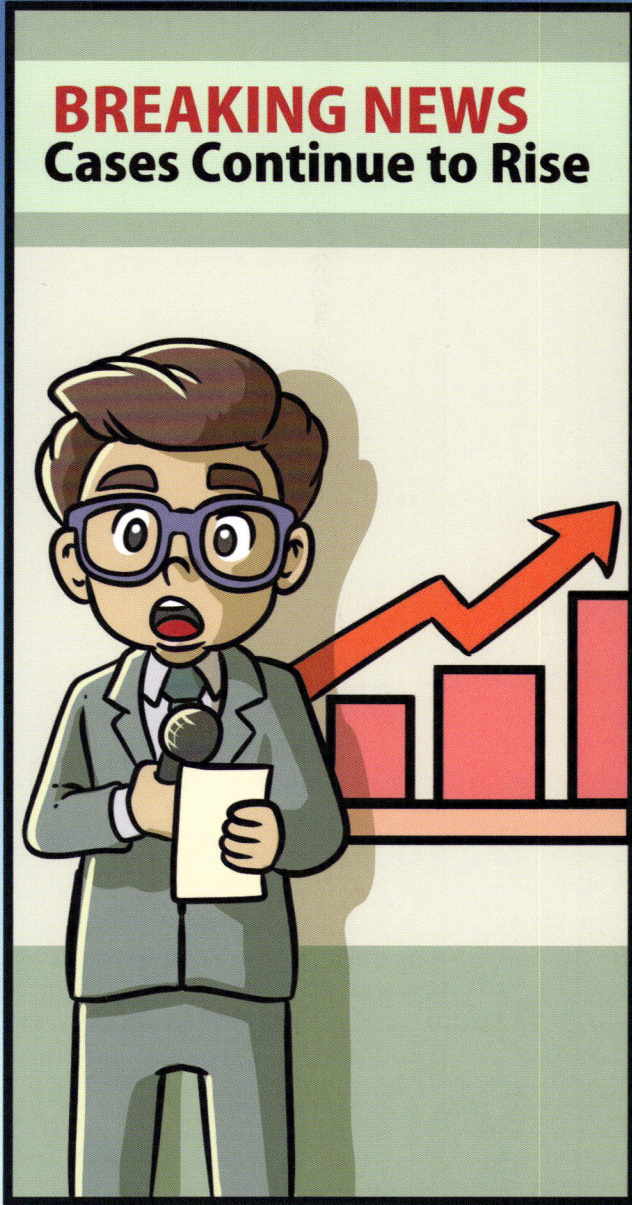

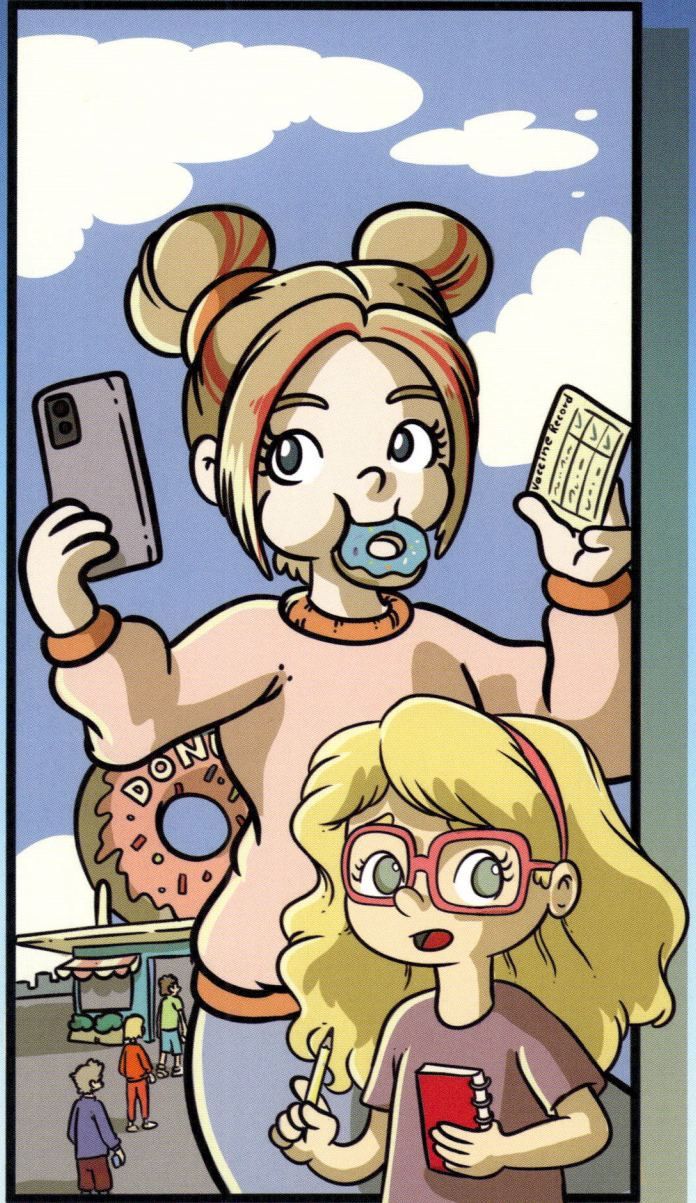

Individuals were even rewarded with donuts, gift cards, money, and other items if they got vaccinated.

All of this is called propaganda.
Let me explain what propaganda means...

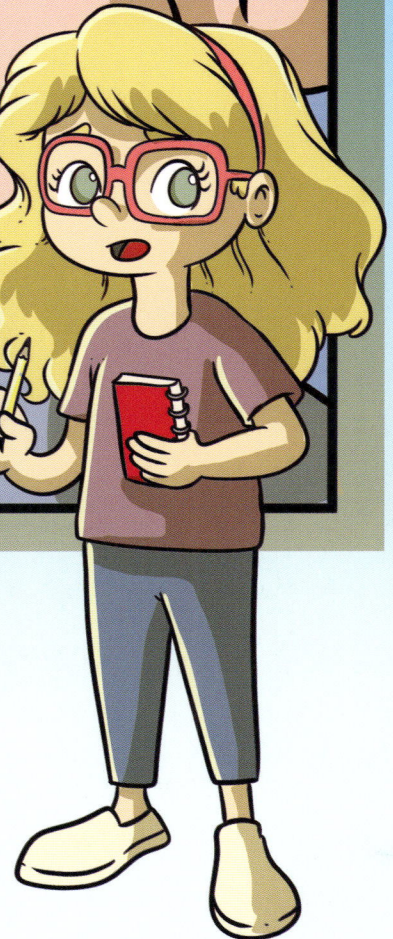

Propaganda is a method of communicating information to make people FEEL a certain way or BELIEVE a certain thing.

Propaganda uses certain words, messages, and powerful images to make people have strong feelings about something, instead of carefully thinking for themselves.

Propaganda can sound negative or positive, as long as it is able to convince people of a certain point of view.

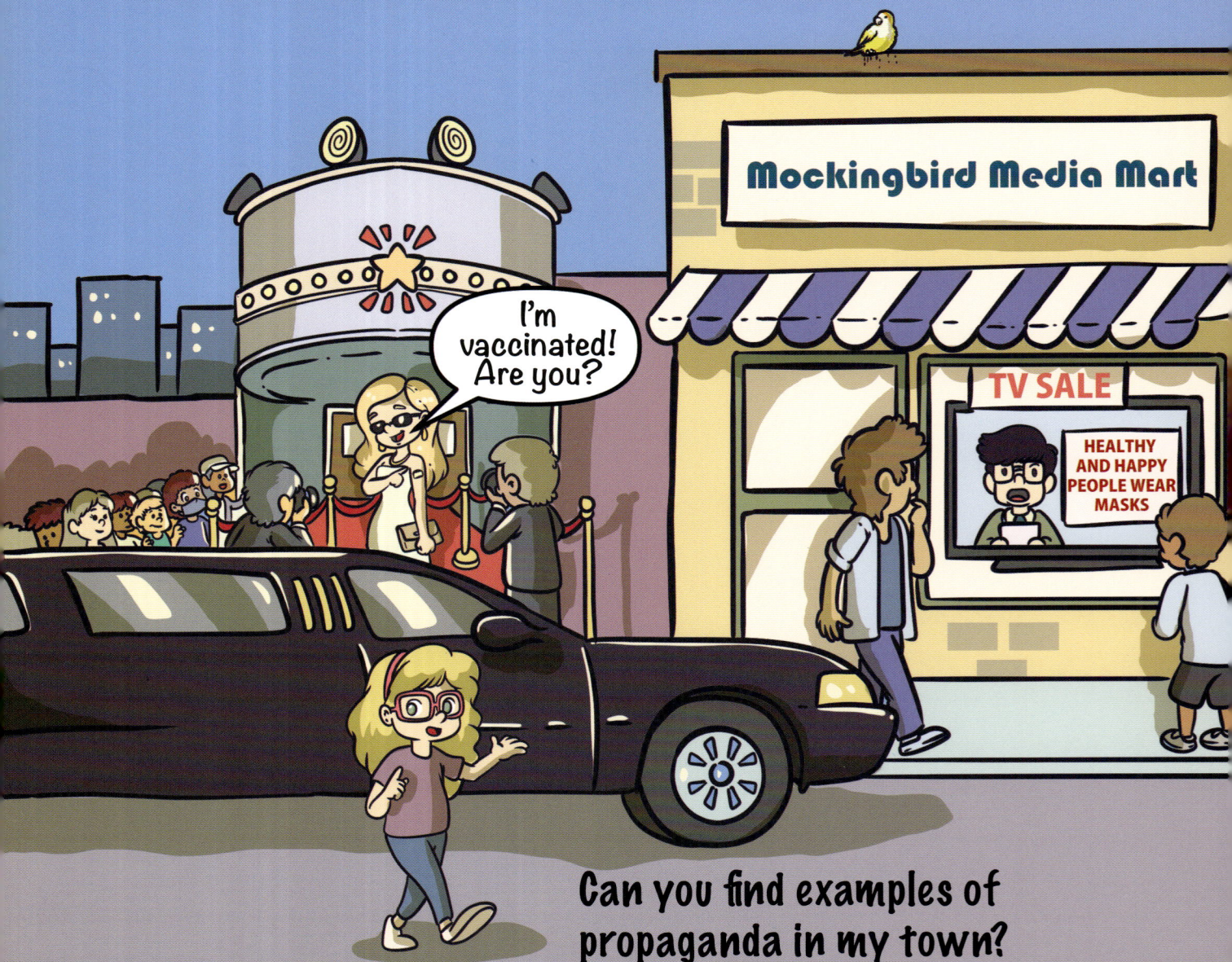

Can you find examples of propaganda in my town?

You may see propaganda on TV commercials, billboards, and anywhere else meant to influence people. Celebrities and politicians often use methods of propaganda to sway opinions.

It's important to know how to spot propaganda so that you can form your own opinions without being told how to think or what to believe.

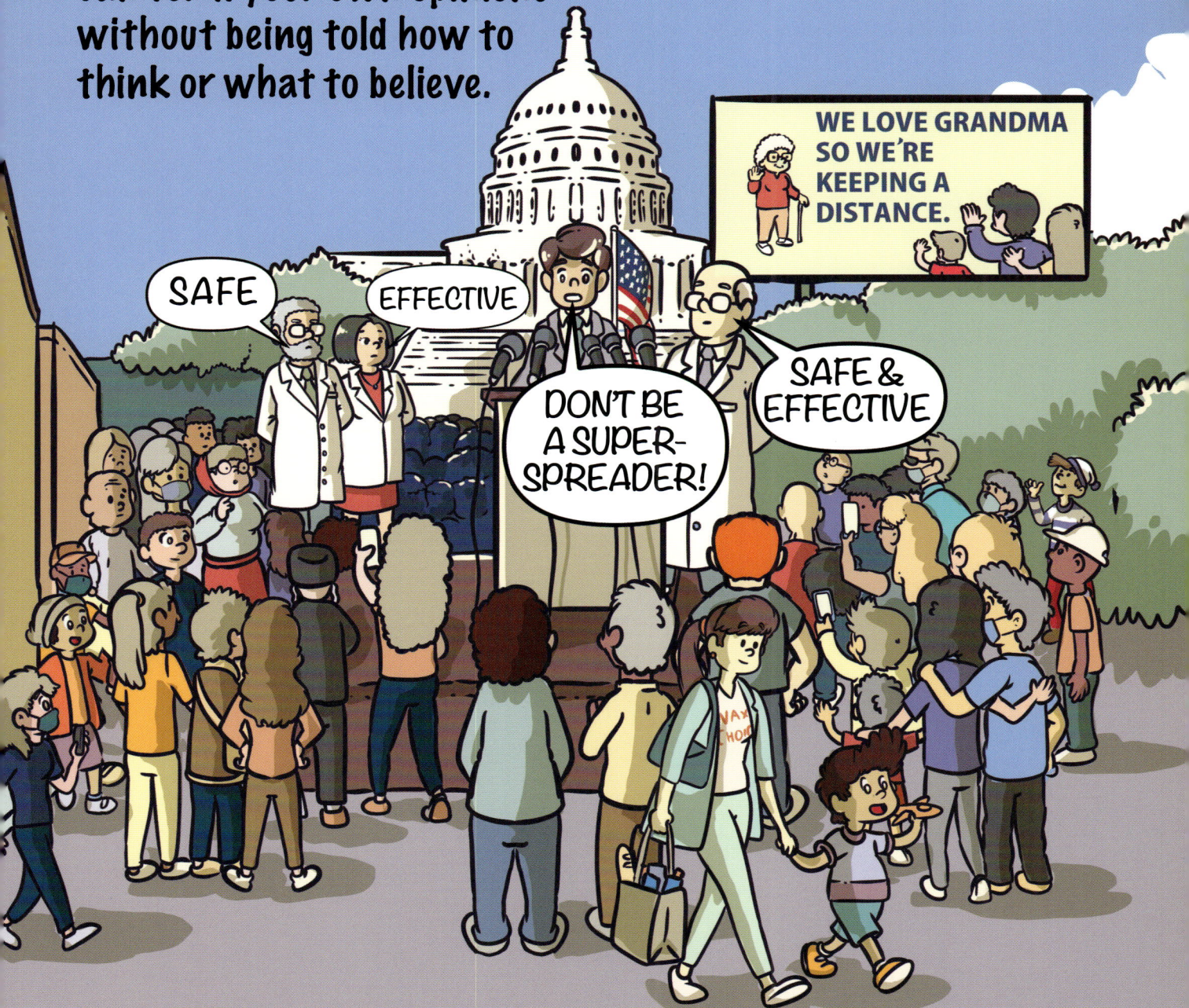

Now that you know a little about propaganda and ways the media and government try to influence people, let's learn how to think critically.

Thinking critically is an important skill that will help you use facts, information, and logic to make educated and informed decisions.

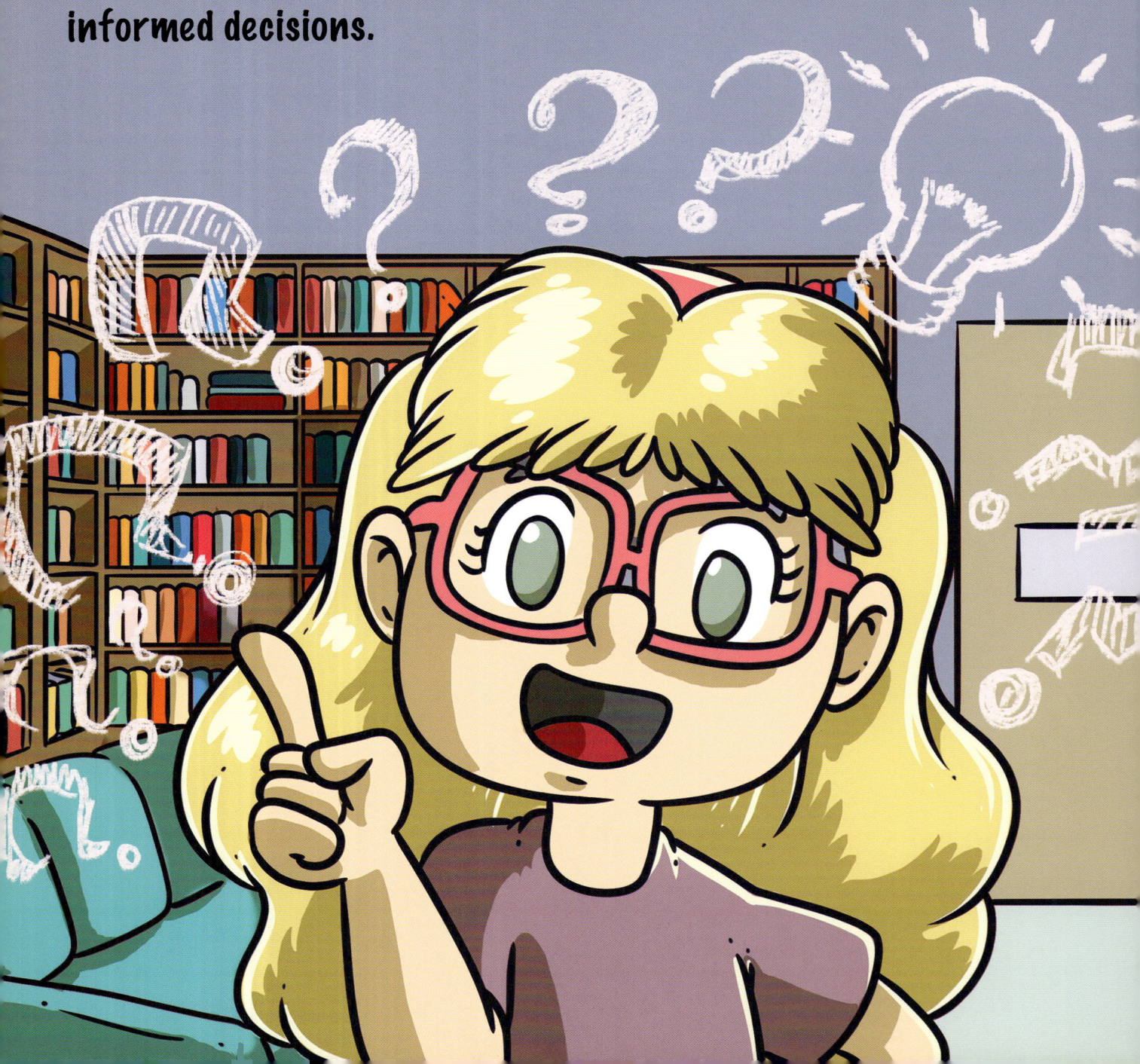

Let's see what my friends say about how to be a good critical thinker.

The first step in critical thinking is knowing what you want to learn about or what you want to discover. This will involve analyzing information, looking at evidence, figuring out the facts, and understanding the arguments.

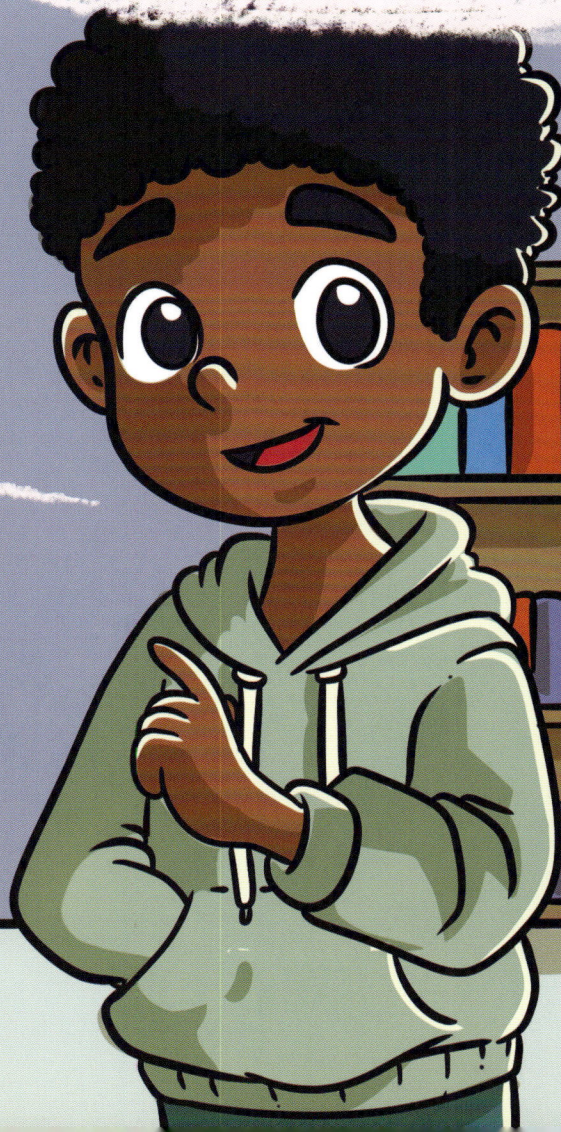

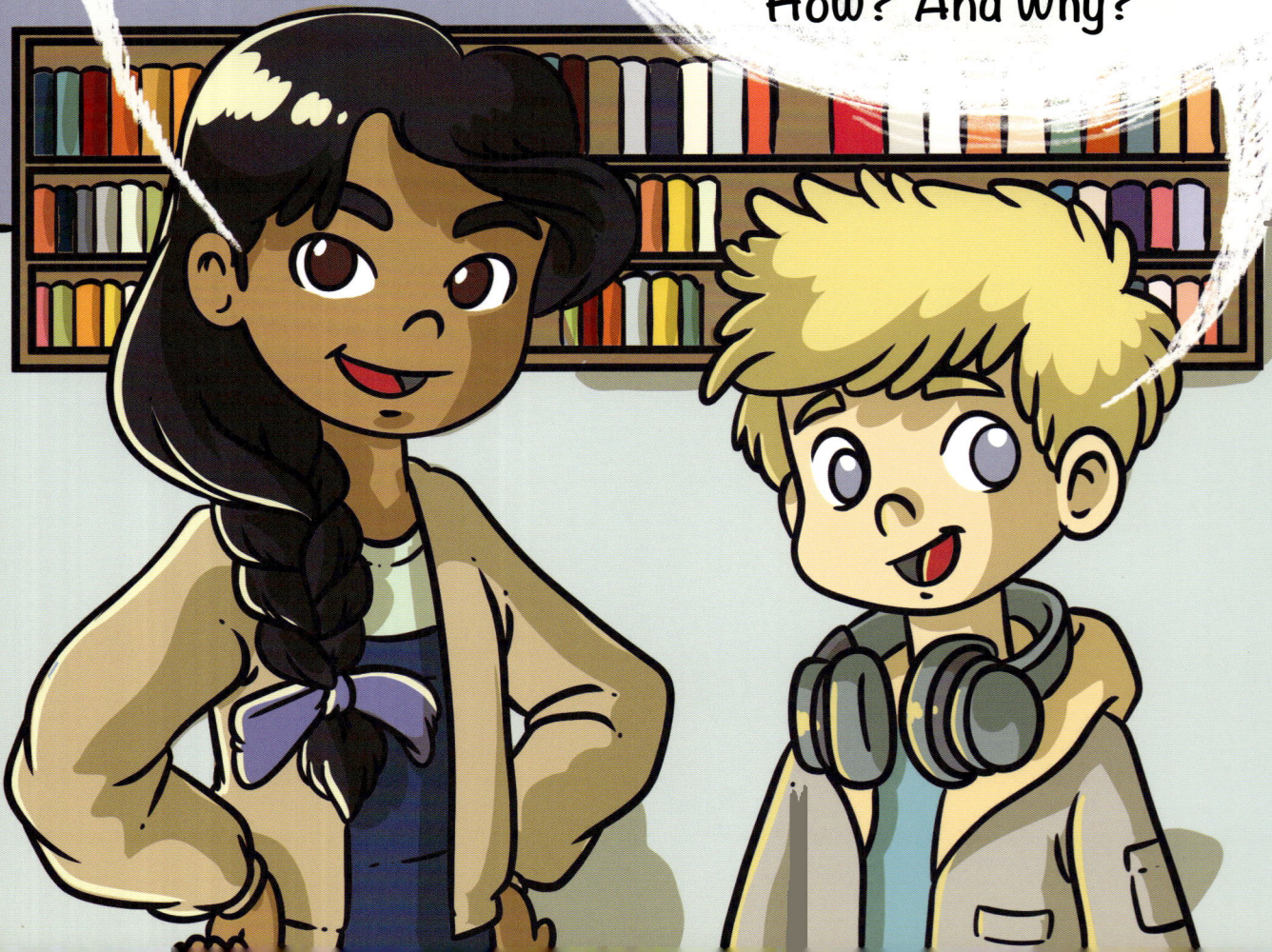

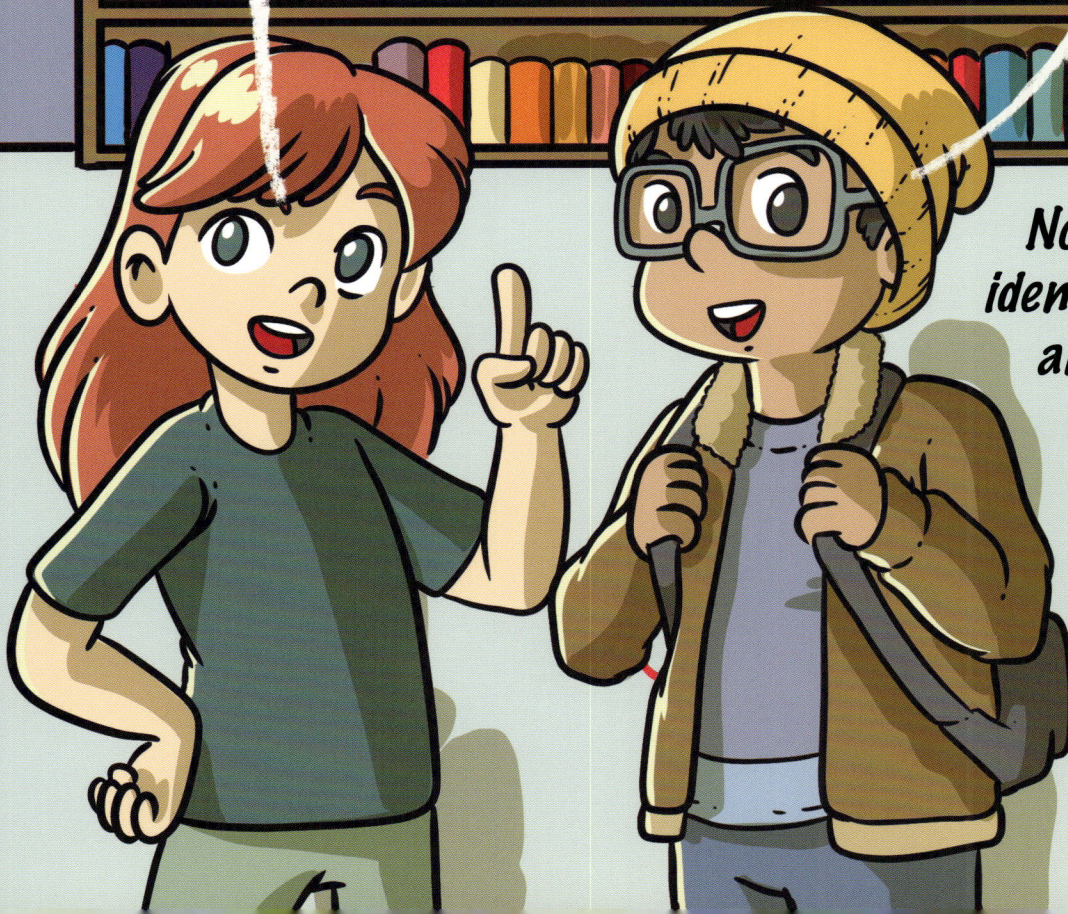

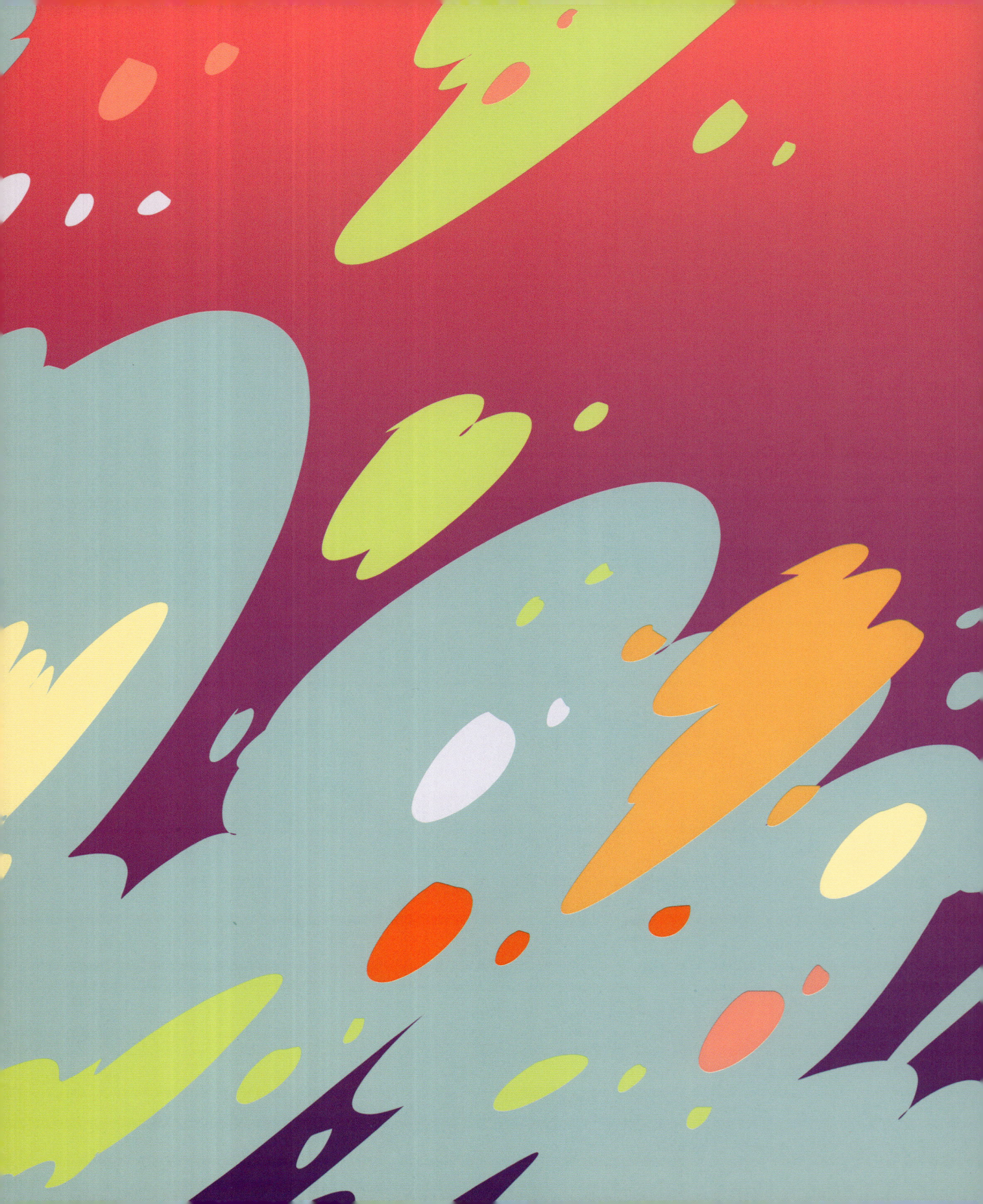

PART TWO:
LET'S INVESTIGATE!
Masks, Lockdowns,
Social Distancing &
Vaccines

During the pandemic, people were told they had to wear masks in public places. The news made many people feel scared by repeating messages over and over from doctors and scientists saying masks would protect us from viruses.

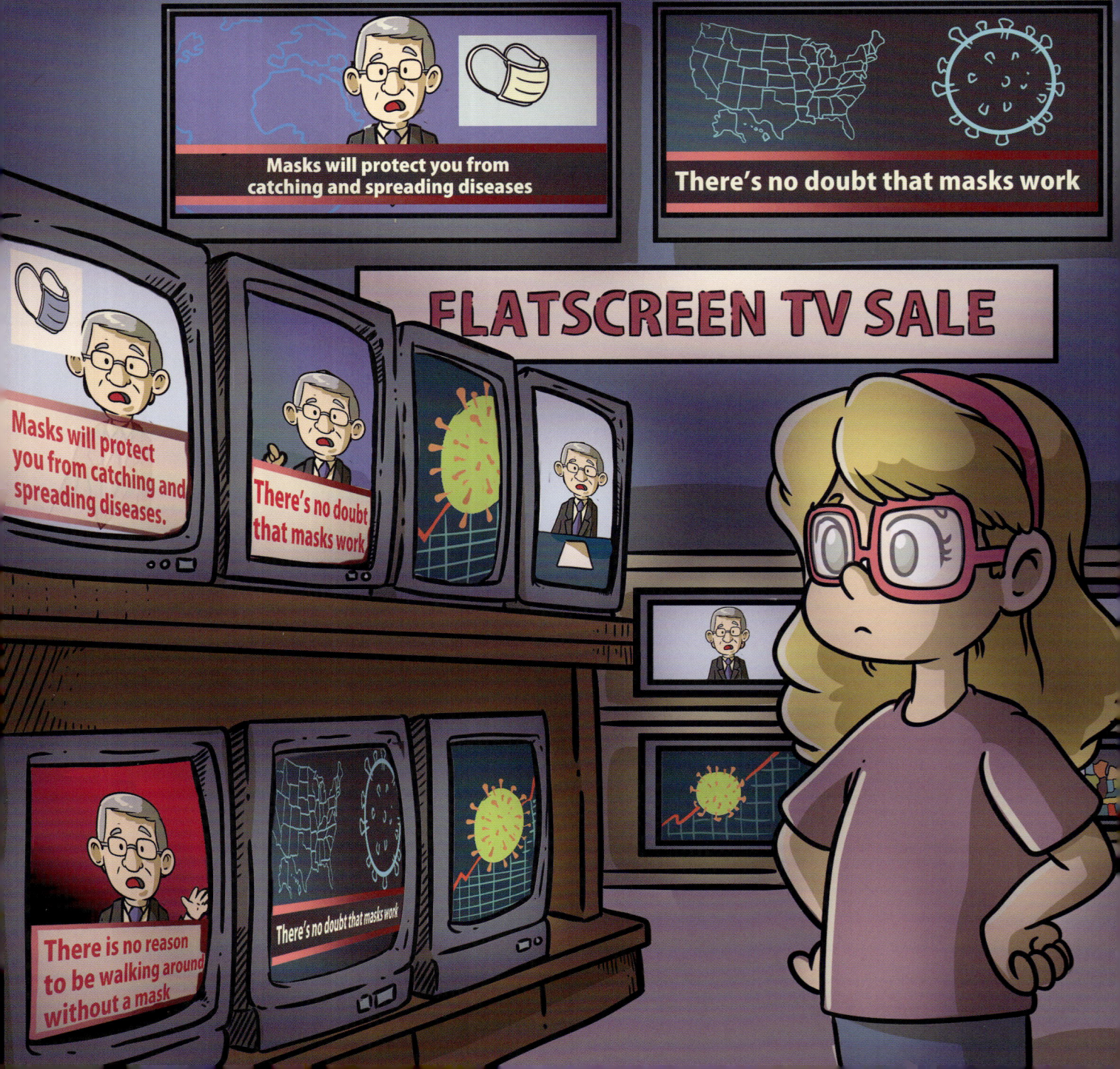

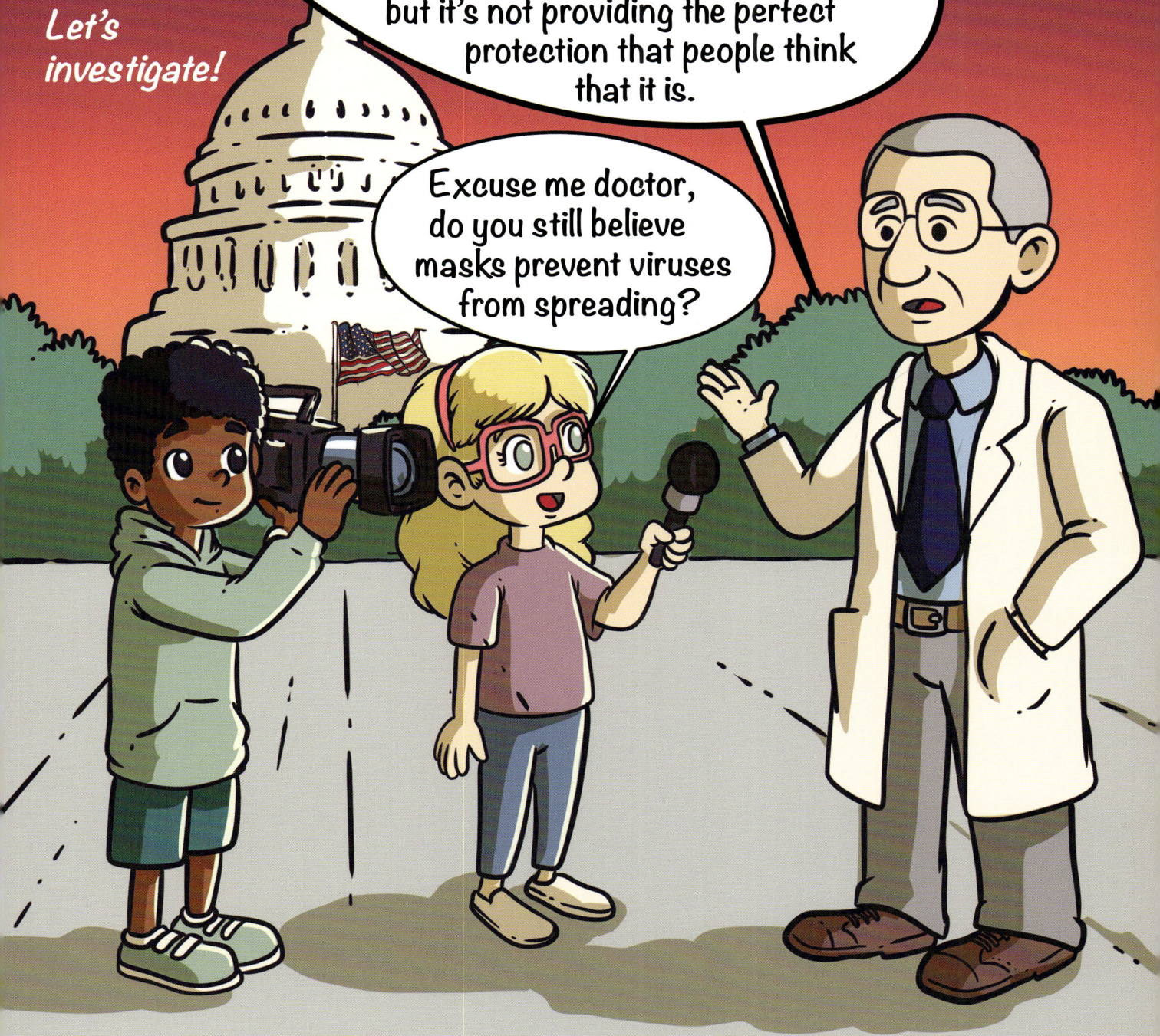

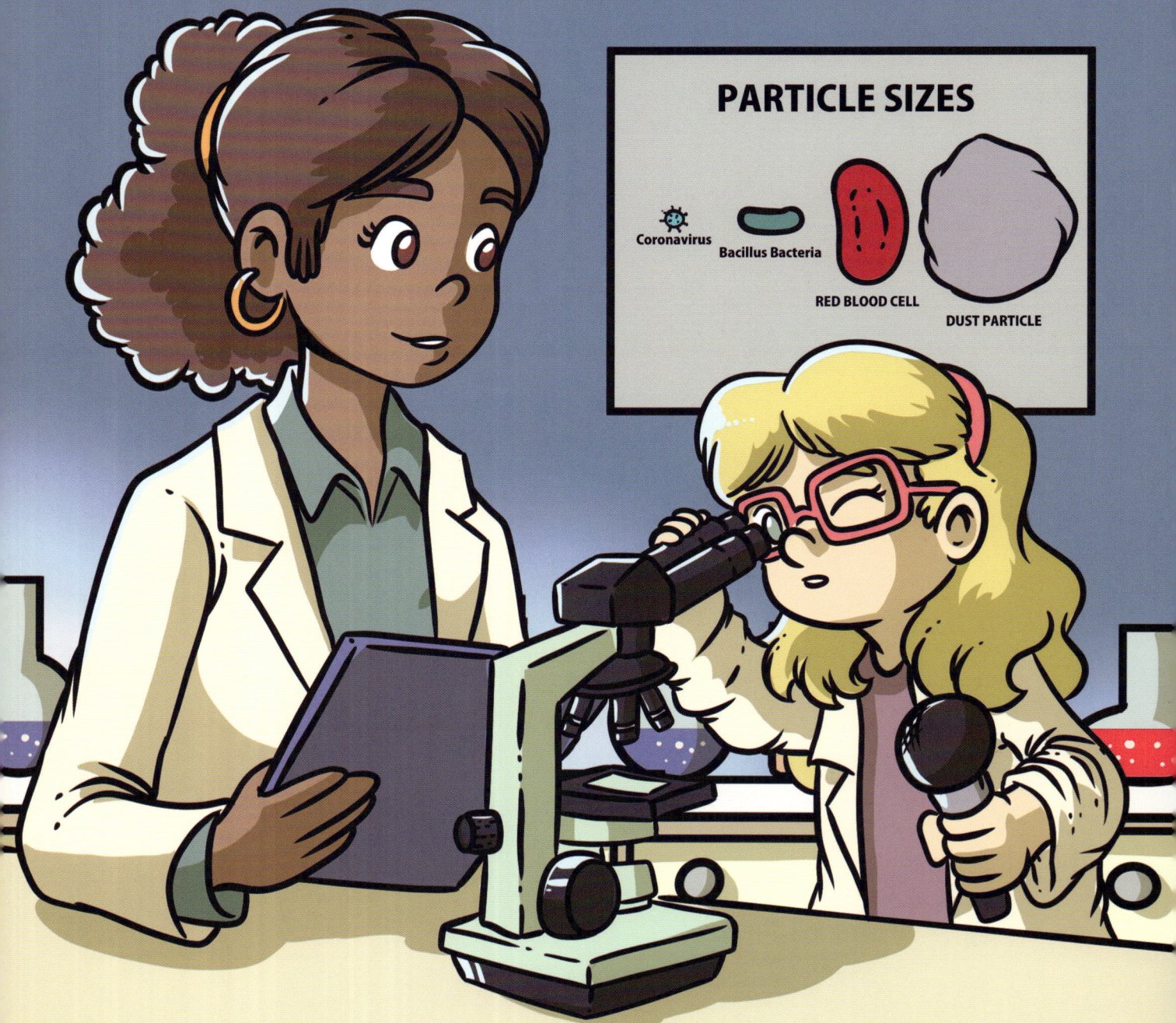

PARTICLE SIZES

Coronavirus

Bacillus Bacteria

RED BLOOD CELL

DUST PARTICLE

To get an even better understanding of masks, and whether they work or not, I interviewed several scientists.

I was surprised to learn that virus particles are so extremely small that they can easily get through your average cloth or paper mask.

During my research, I also discovered that people who wear masks often speak louder and pronounce their words clearer because they want to be heard and understood.

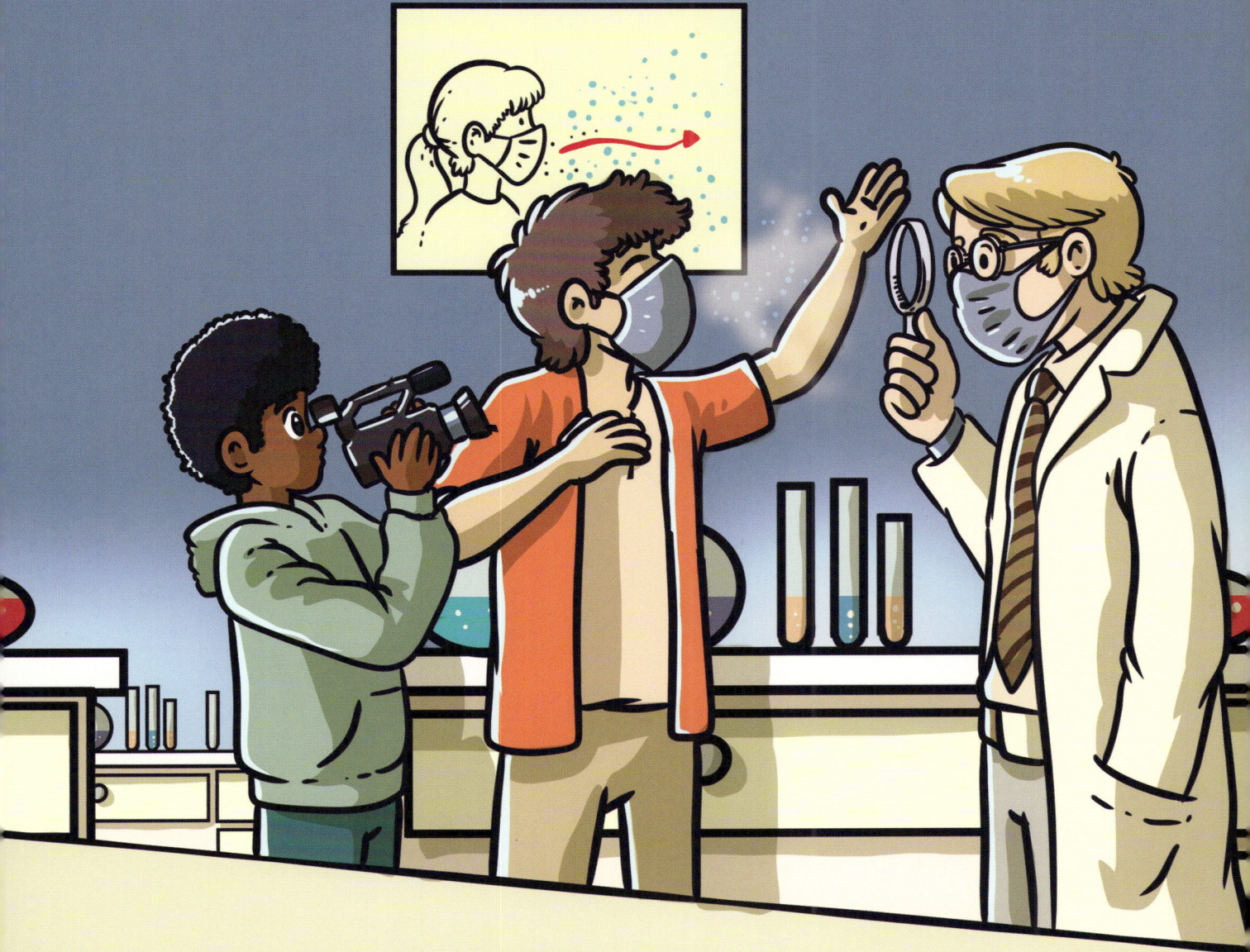

These scientists explained that speaking louder and pronouncing words clearer causes more saliva particles to be sprayed outward, making it easier to spread germs.

Critical thinking challenge: Based on what you've learned about masks, do you think masks work at blocking germs?

SCHOOL LOCKDOWNS

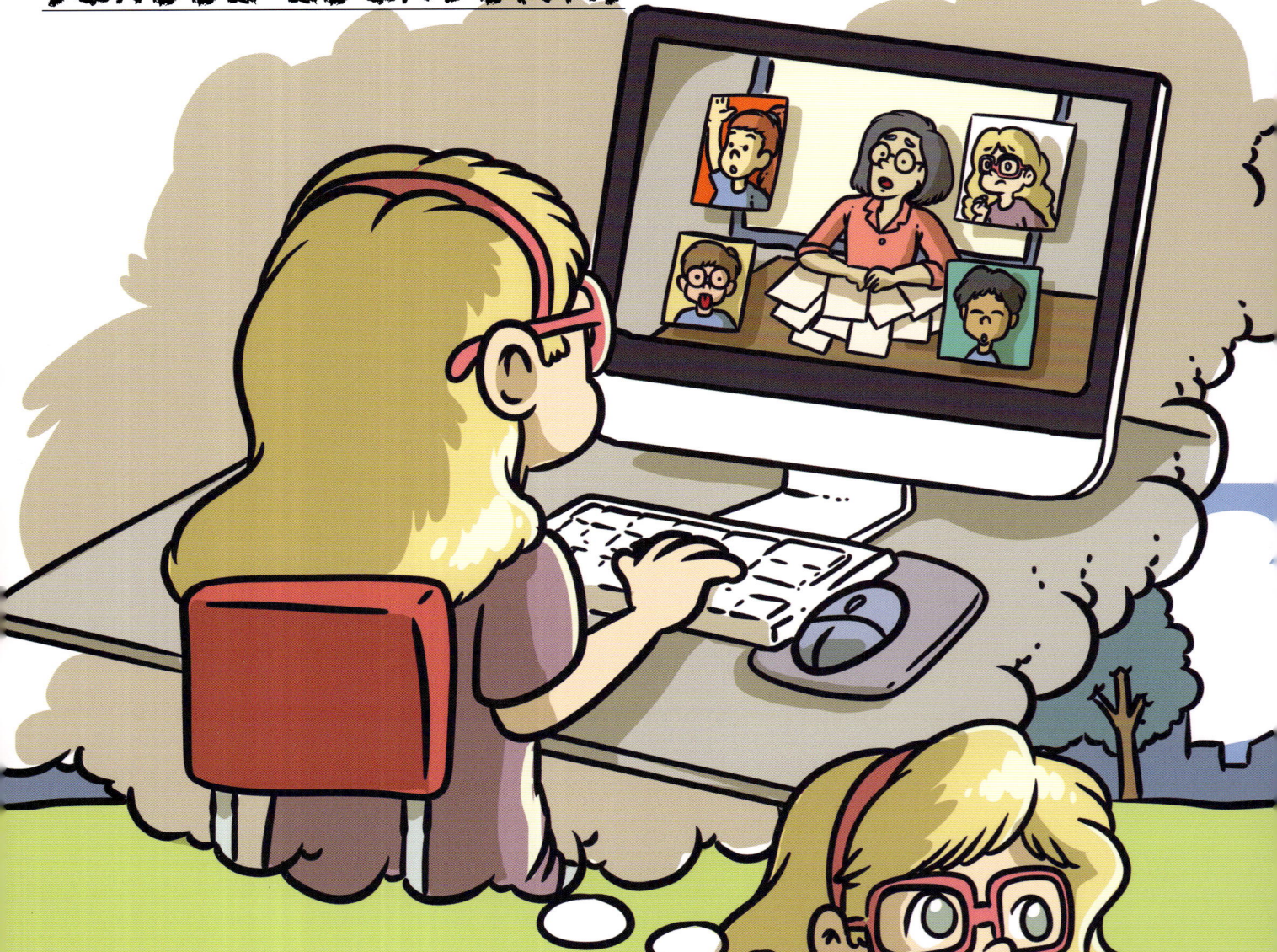

School is very important to me. I love my friends, teachers, and learning new things.

When the pandemic happened, and schools "locked down," many of my classmates had a difficult time. Suddenly, we had to attend school online. For many of us, online school became a daily struggle.

How did you handle school during the pandemic?

As part of my investigative research, I asked my friends about their own school experience during the pandemic.

I wondered how they handled the sudden change in school from in-person to online and wanted to know if they struggled with the lockdowns like I did. Let's investigate!

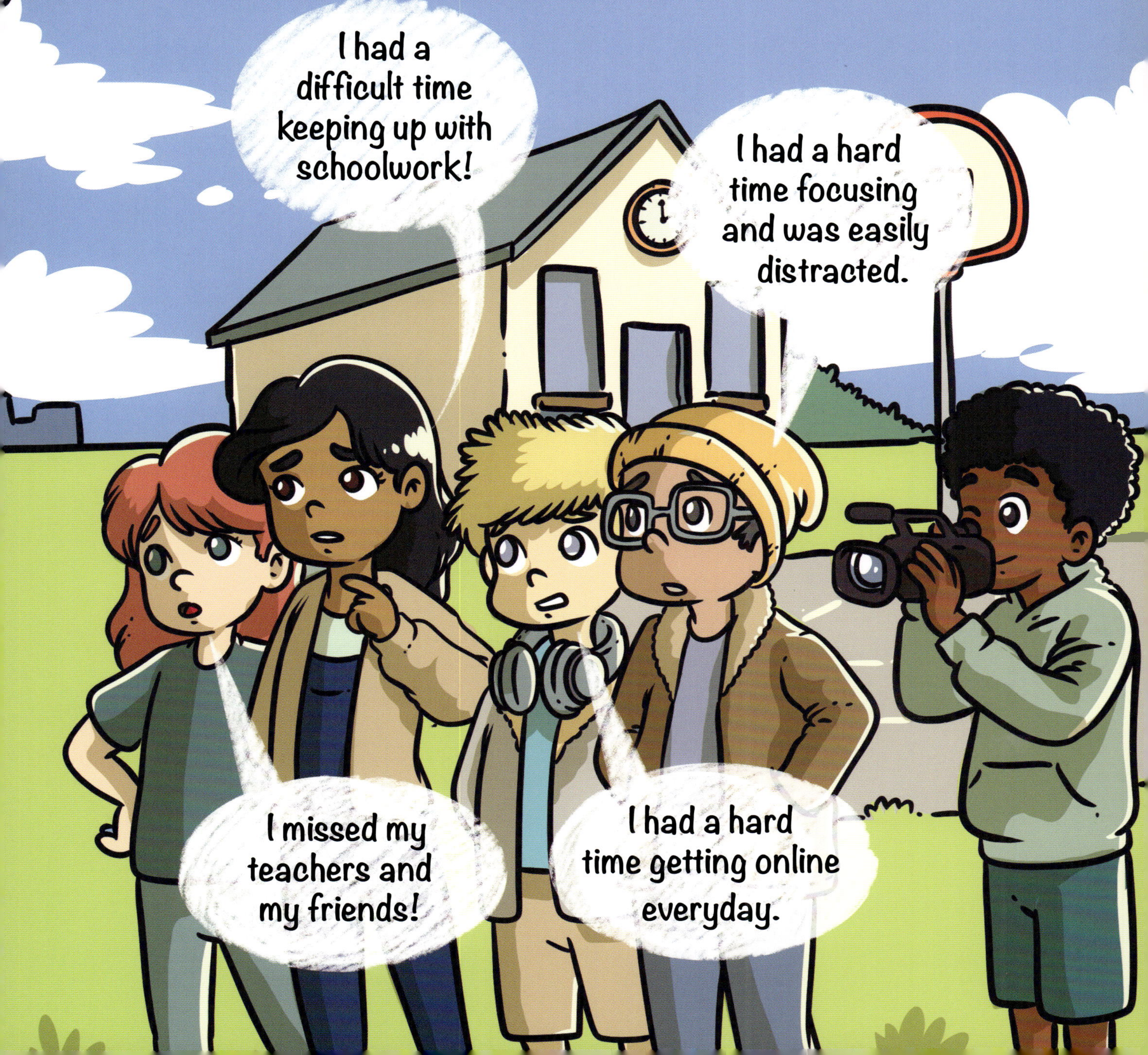

SCHOOL LOCKDOWNS continued

Since many kids my age had a difficult time with school lockdowns, I decided to speak with a psychologist to learn more about the effects lockdowns had on students.

Psychologists are doctors who understand different human emotions and behaviors.

Based on your own experience, what did you discover about school lockdowns and how they affected kids my age?

Some psychologists help people get through hard times in their lives, while other psychologists spend their time researching the way people feel and behave.

Critical Thinking Challenge: Based on what you've learned about school lockdowns, were they more helpful or hurtful to students?

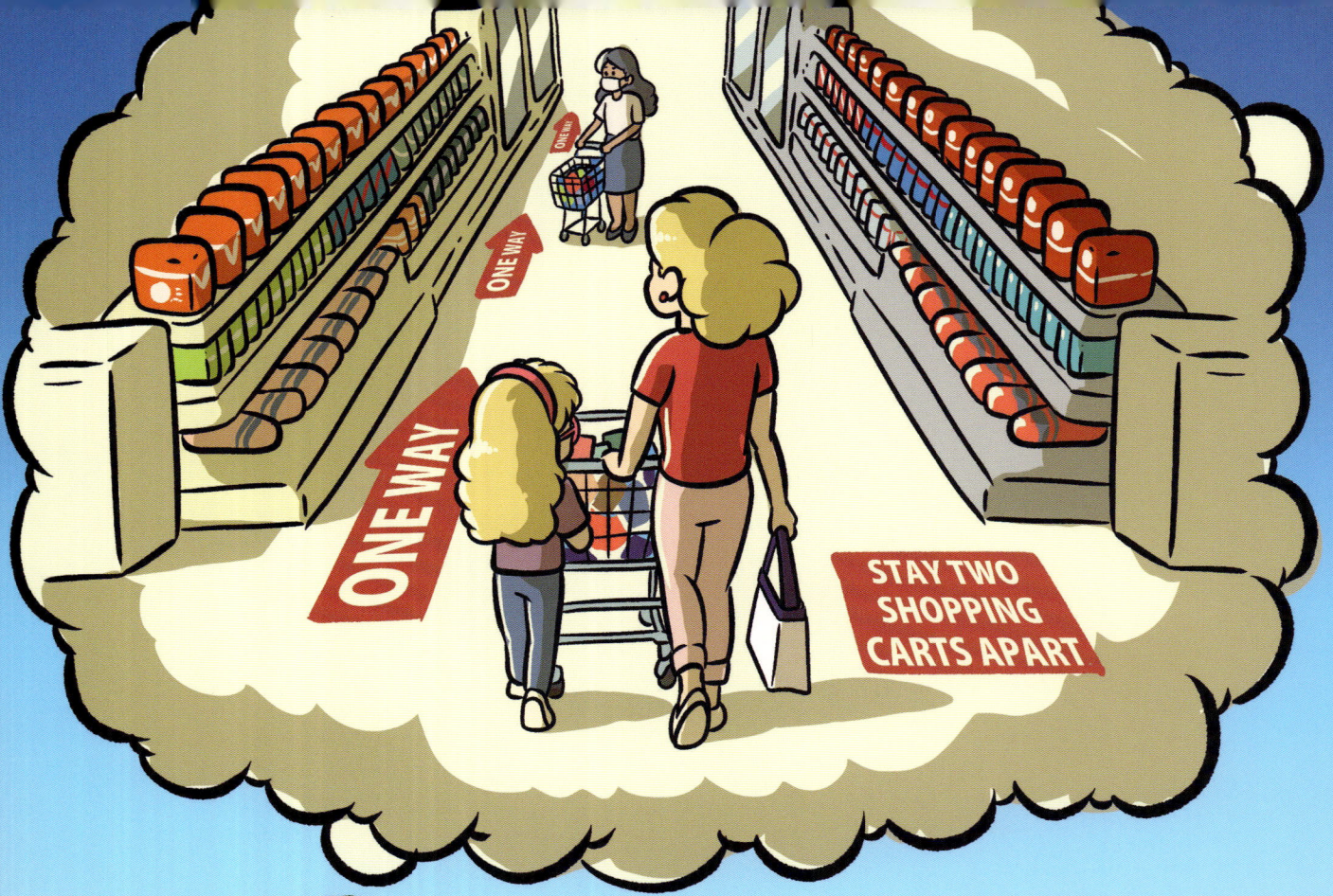

SOCIAL DISTANCING: The six-foot rule

During the pandemic, people were told to stay six feet away from each other as another way to stay safe.

This was called social distancing.

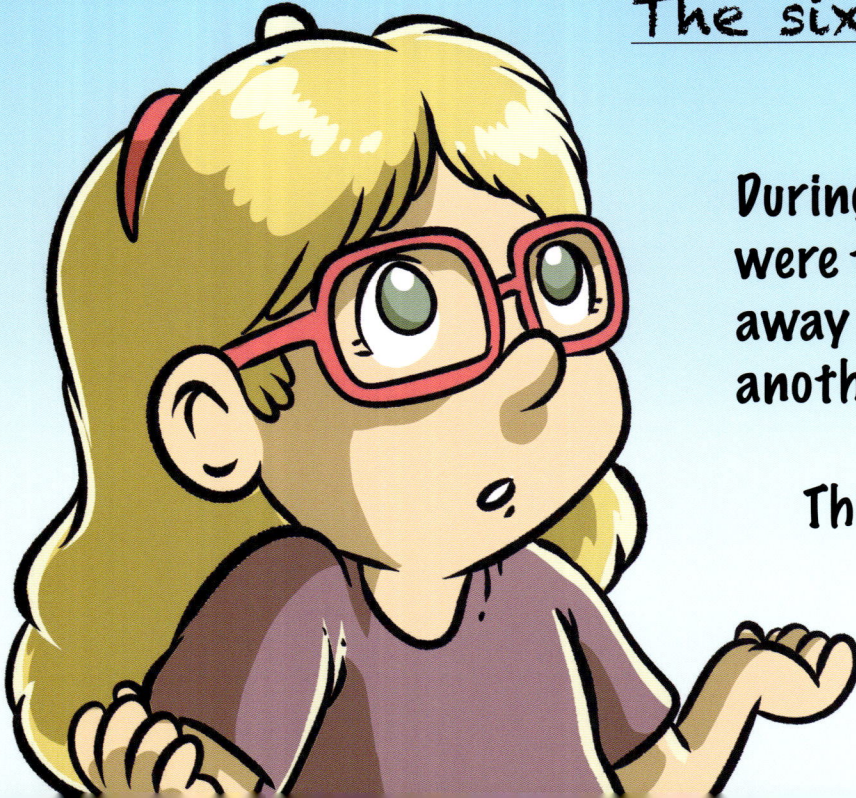

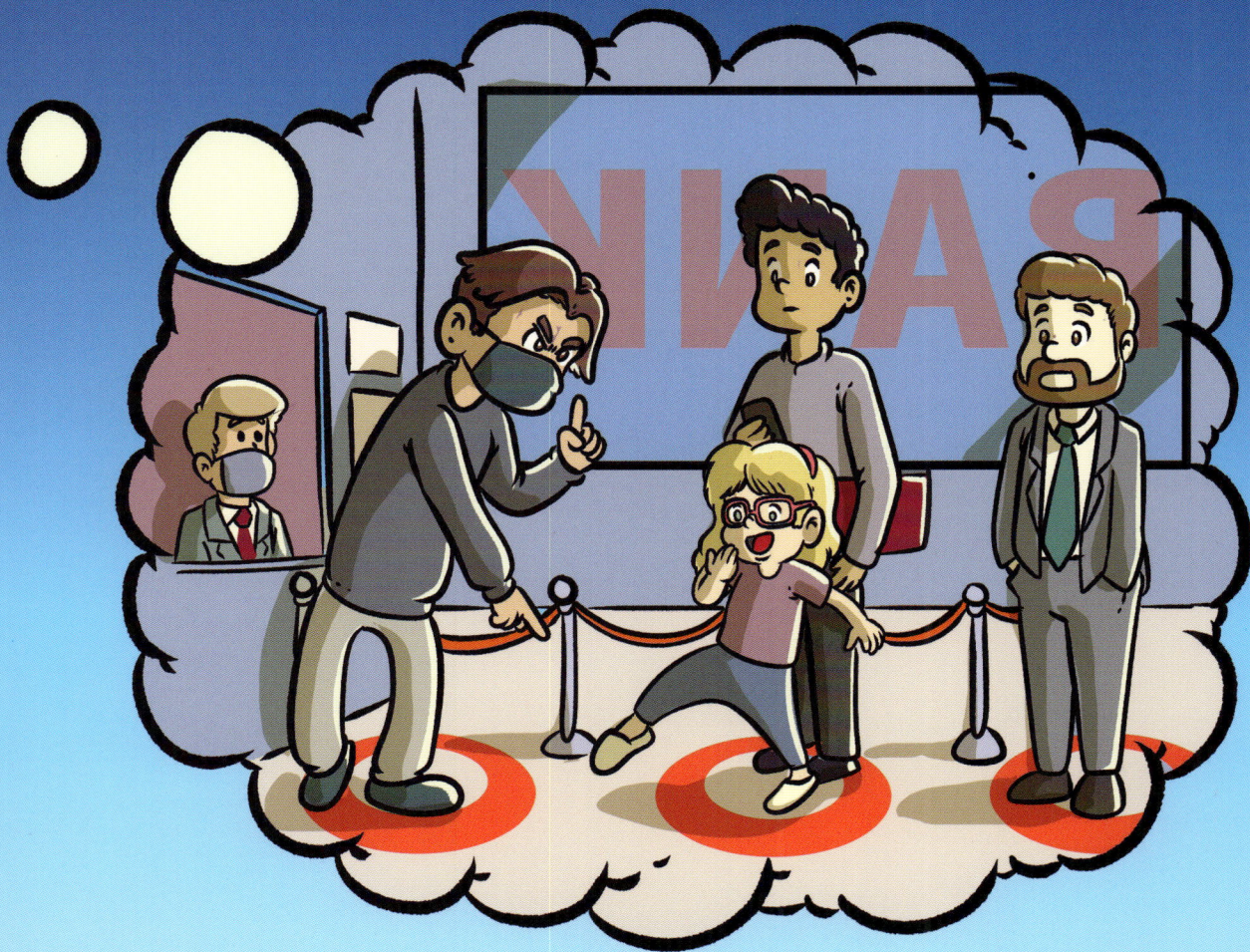

This six-foot rule for social distancing was used in most public places. Many businesses had stickers on the floor, telling people which direction to walk and where to stand.

Originally, the six-foot rule was created because scientists believed germs from coughs and sneezes could only travel up to six feet away and make people sick.

But, if germs travel through the air, why would they stop at six feet? Wouldn't they just keep floating from everyone and go everywhere? This rule just never made sense to me.
Let's investigate!

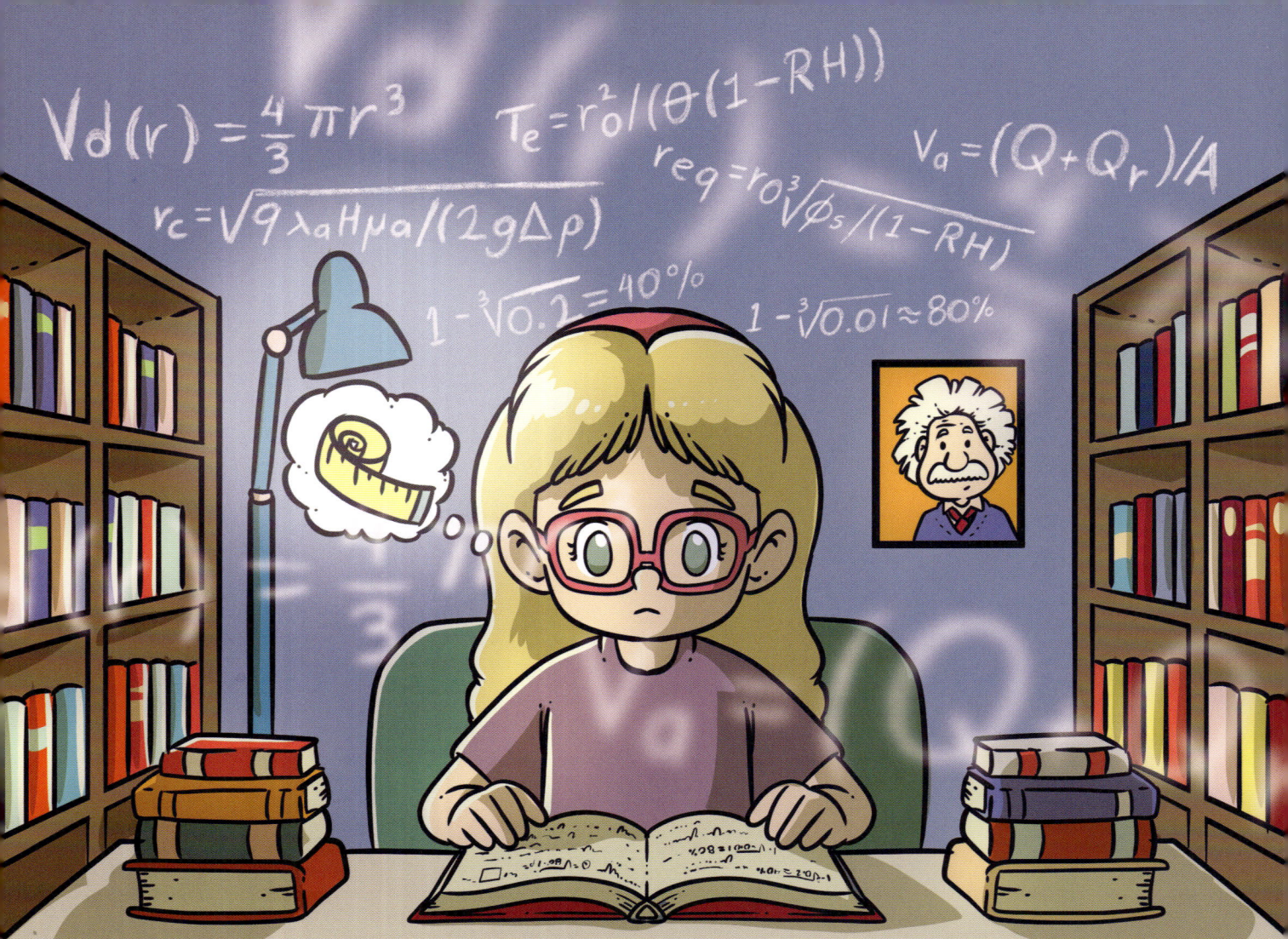

SOCIAL DISTANCING continued

To learn more about social distancing, I read a study where scientists looked at how droplets of saliva move through the air when people talk, sneeze, sing, or breathe. These scientists used math to measure if staying six feet apart really stopped germs from spreading. Their research found that germs can travel much farther than six feet—sometimes even up to sixty feet, depending on how many people are in a room or if the room has open windows for air to move around.

This was great information, but I still wanted to learn more.

Next, I went to an important meeting in Washington, DC, where politicians spoke about the rules that were made during the pandemic. During this meeting, I discovered that social distancing guidelines were never based on scientific research!

Critical thinking challenge: Based on what you've learned about social distancing, did the six-foot rule help protect people from exposure to germs?

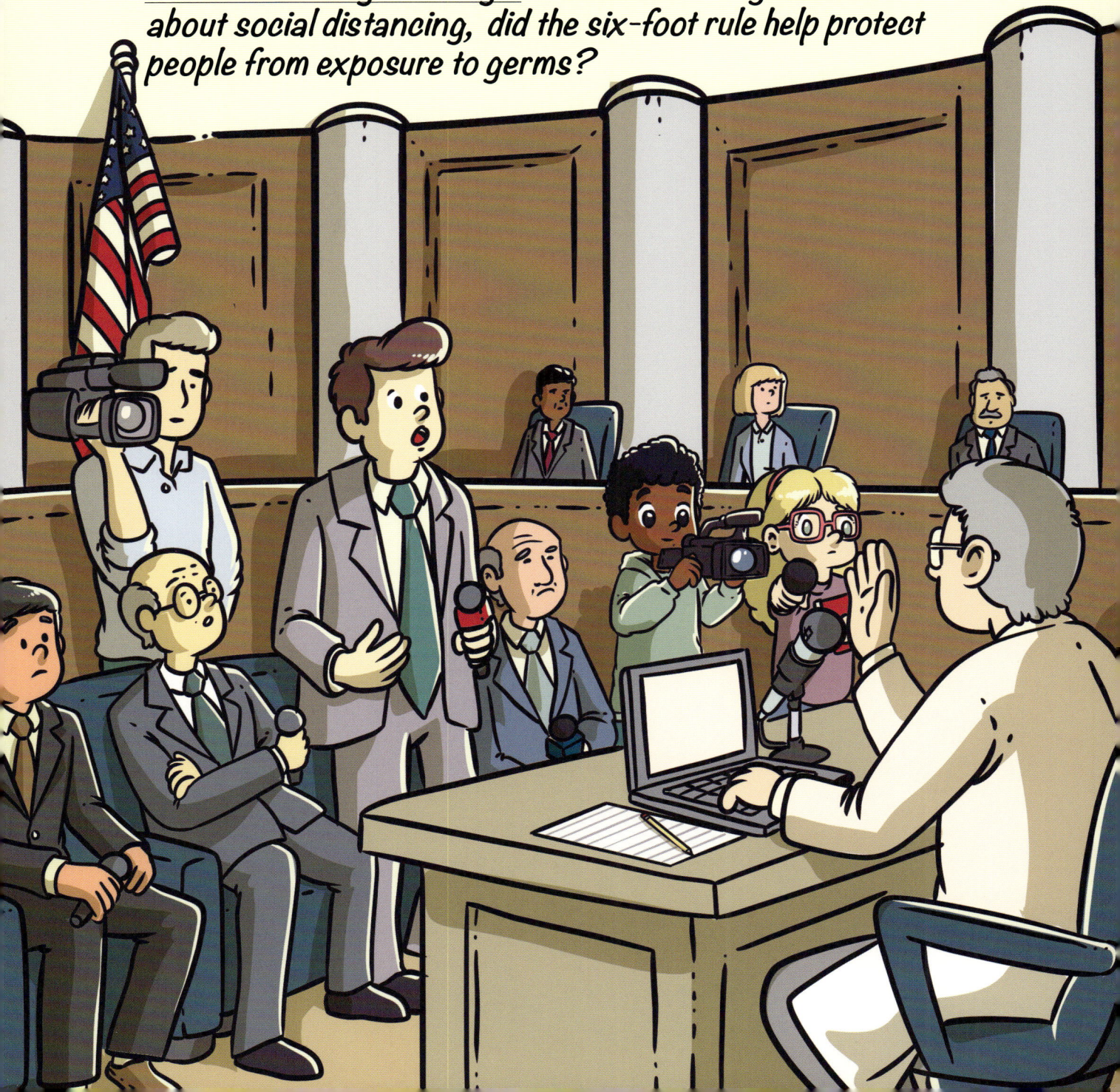

VACCINES

Vaccines have been debated for a very long time. Even though the news, politicians, vaccine makers, and many doctors say that vaccines are safe, most people still want to be sure that shots won't harm them.

During the pandemic, vaccines were produced very quickly while much of the world was panicking. These shots were made using a new mRNA technology, causing some people to further question their safety. Yet, without any long-term safety studies, vaccines were mandated for most Americans! This vaccine mandate meant that shots were required for school and work.

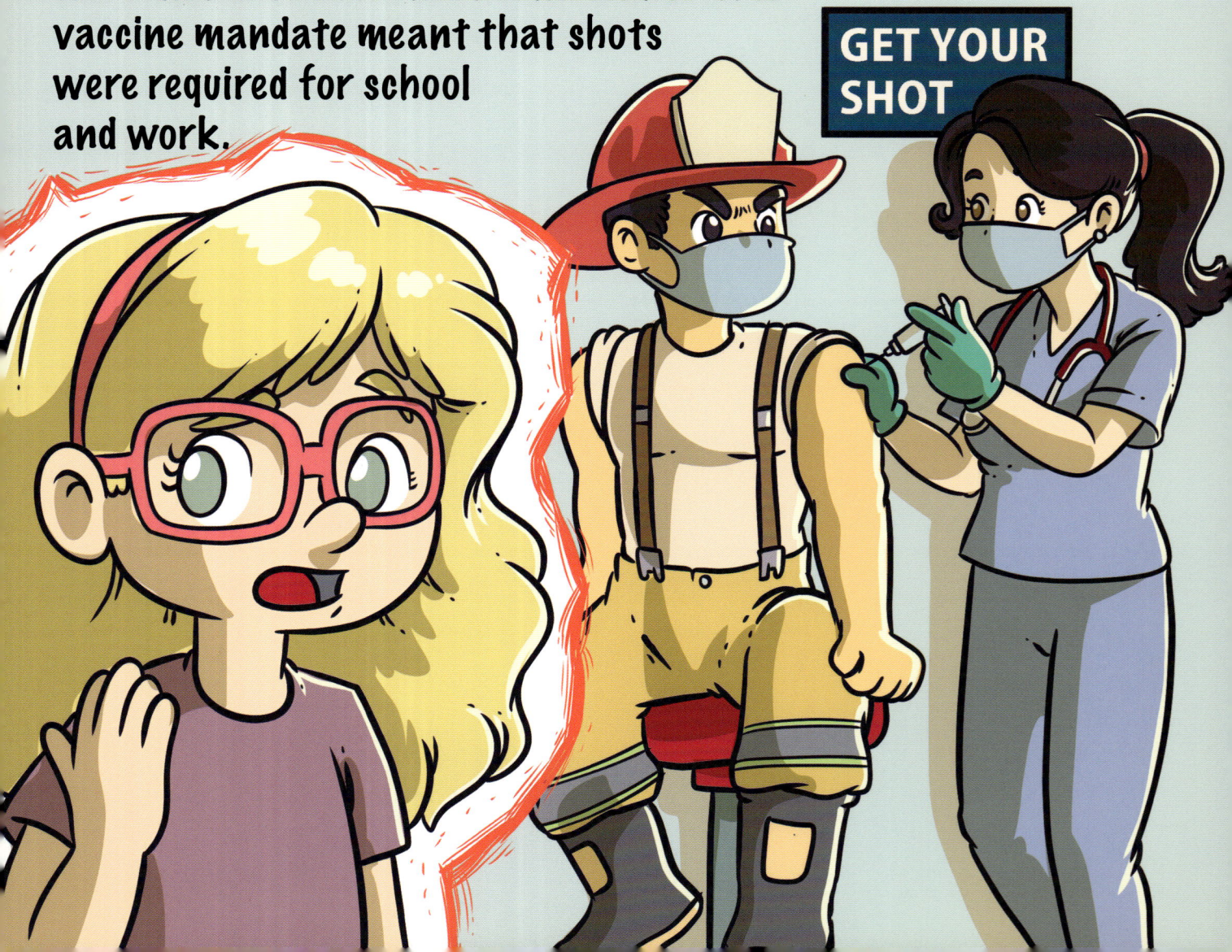

GET YOUR SHOT

The mandate caused many people to get vaccinated, even though they may not have wanted to. Sadly, many ended up very sick or permanently injured following these forced shots. It also denied people true informed consent. This means they weren't given all the information about possible dangers, so they couldn't make an informed choice before receiving the shot.

So, are mRNA vaccines actually safe? Let's investigate!

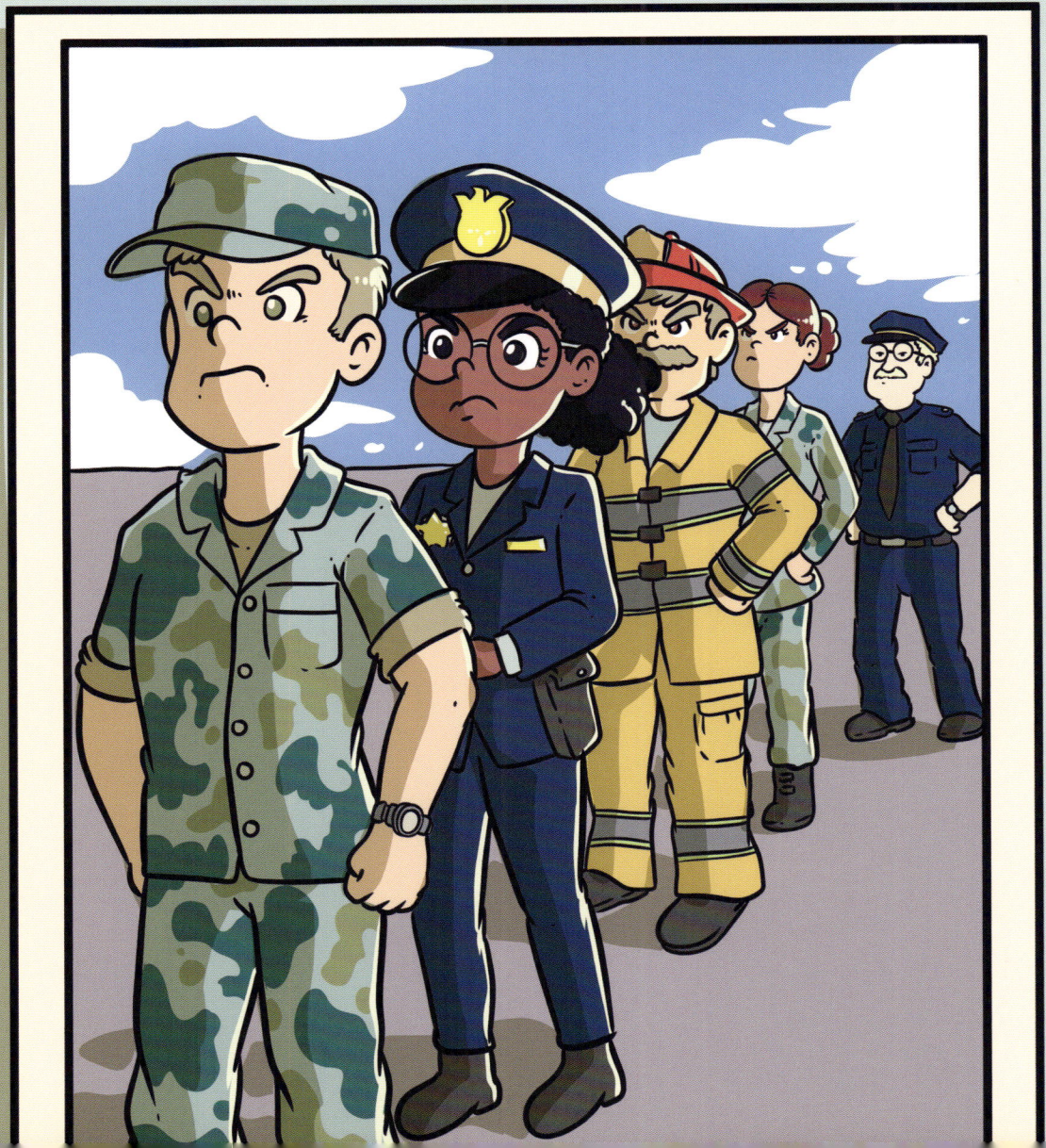

VACCINES SAVE LIVES

PROTECTING THOSE WHO PROTECT US

VACCINES continued

For this research, I spoke directly with a surgeon general to get his opinion on the safety of mRNA vaccines.

A surgeon general is someone appointed by the government to be an official spokesperson on public health matters.

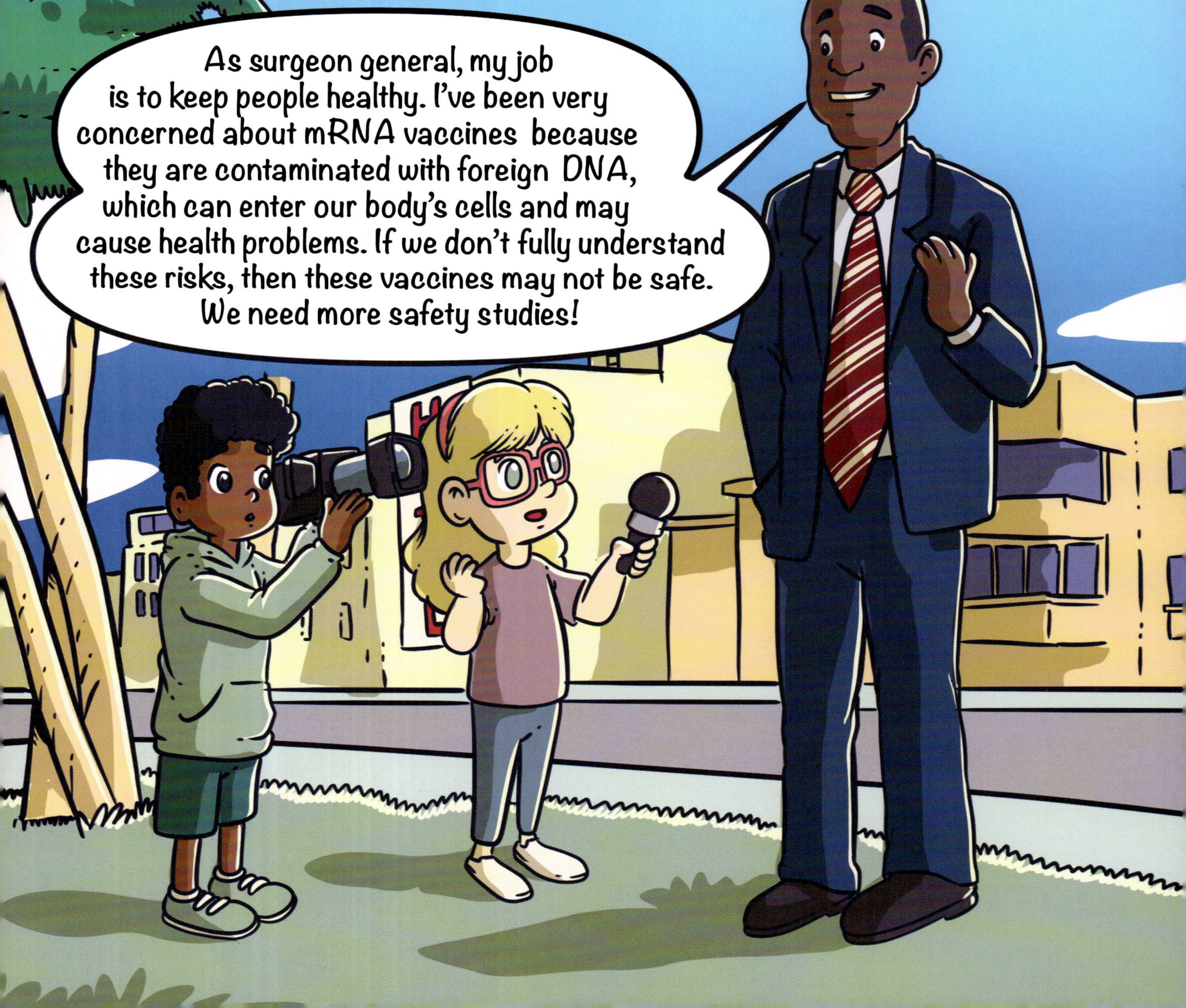

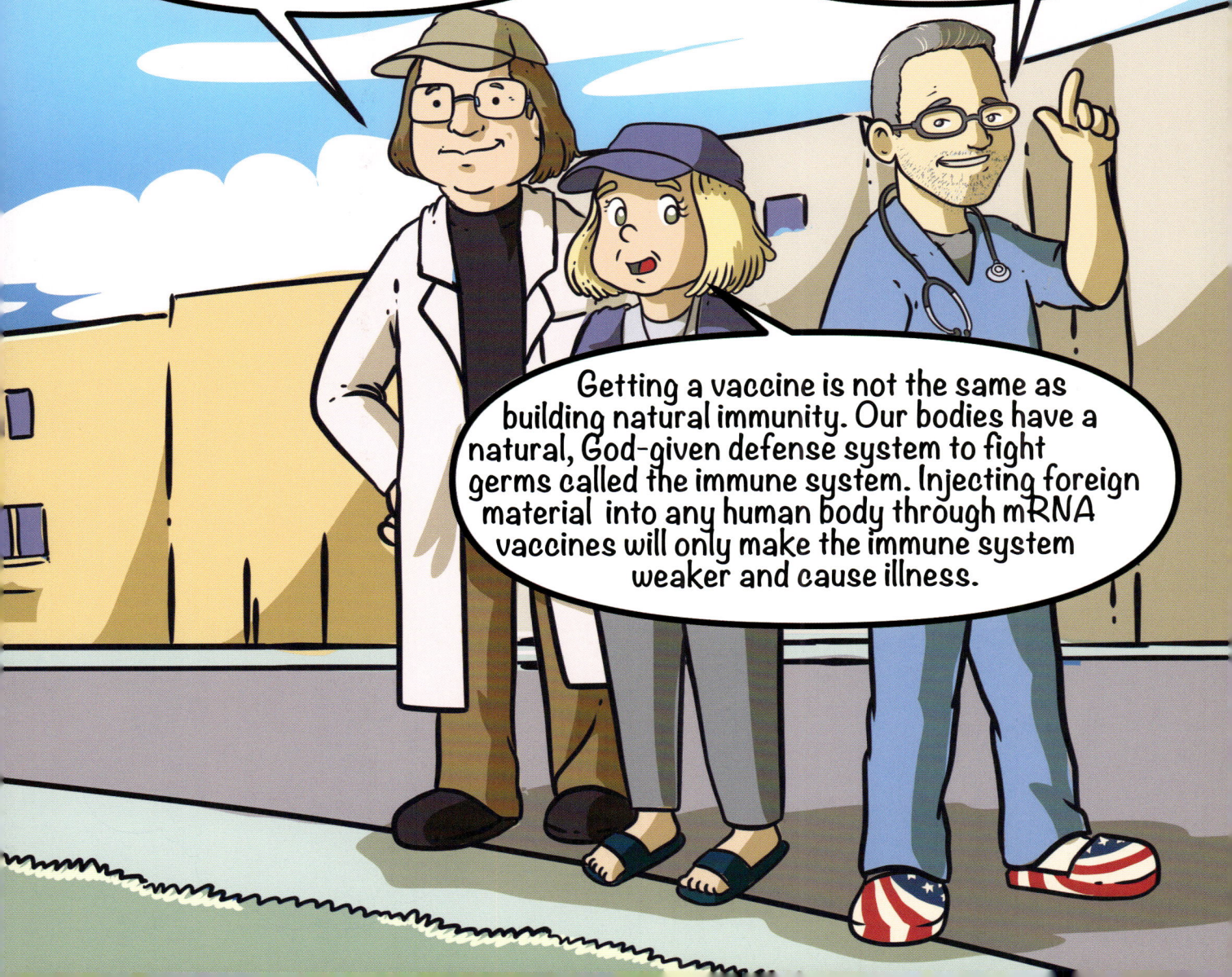

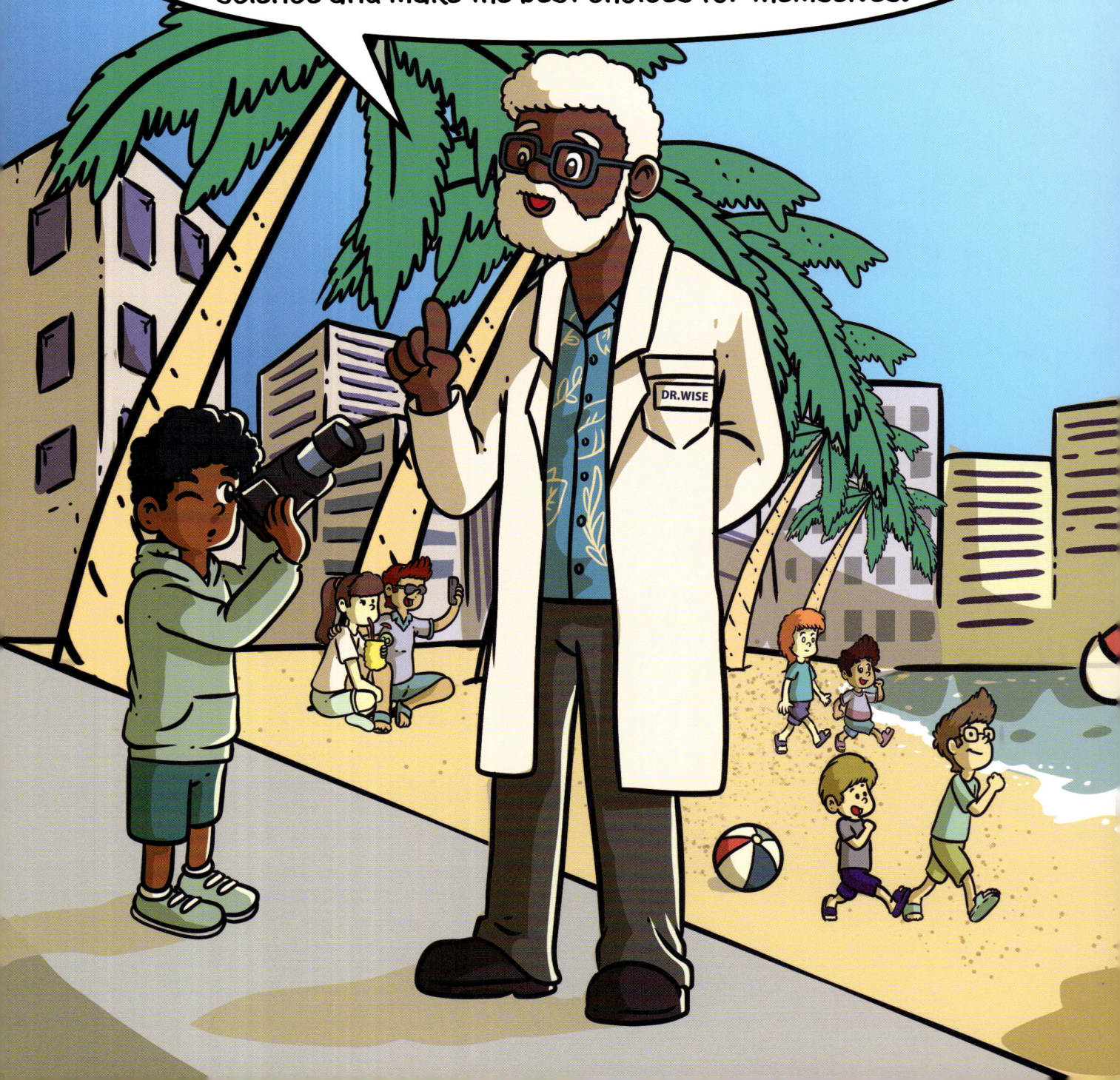

When scientists and doctors have different opinions in science, sometimes important information gets hidden on purpose. This is called censorship.

Censorship is when certain ideas or messages are blocked from being shared and seen by the public because the messages don't align with the information the government wants you to have.

Censorship is a serious problem because new ideas help us to learn and grow. If we are unable to hear all sides, it's harder for people to make smart choices about their health. We must always let scientists and doctors share what they know so everyone has the opportunity to learn all the facts, even if we personally disagree with the information.

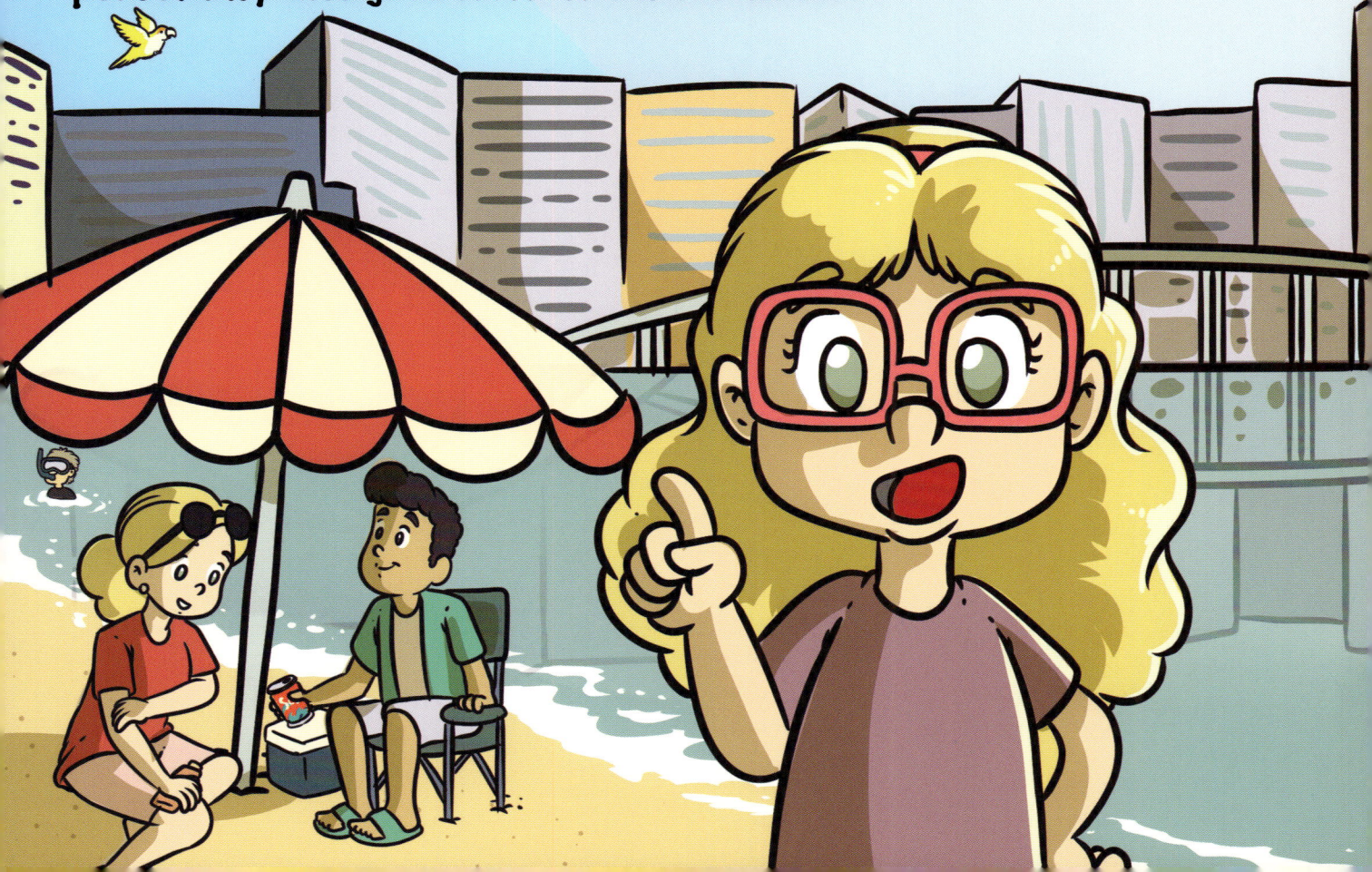

Science is always changing. As more research is done, more information is discovered. It's important that we know how to understand this information so we can form our own opinions and beliefs.

Learning how to recognize propaganda and fact-check our sources will help us make the best decisions for ourselves.

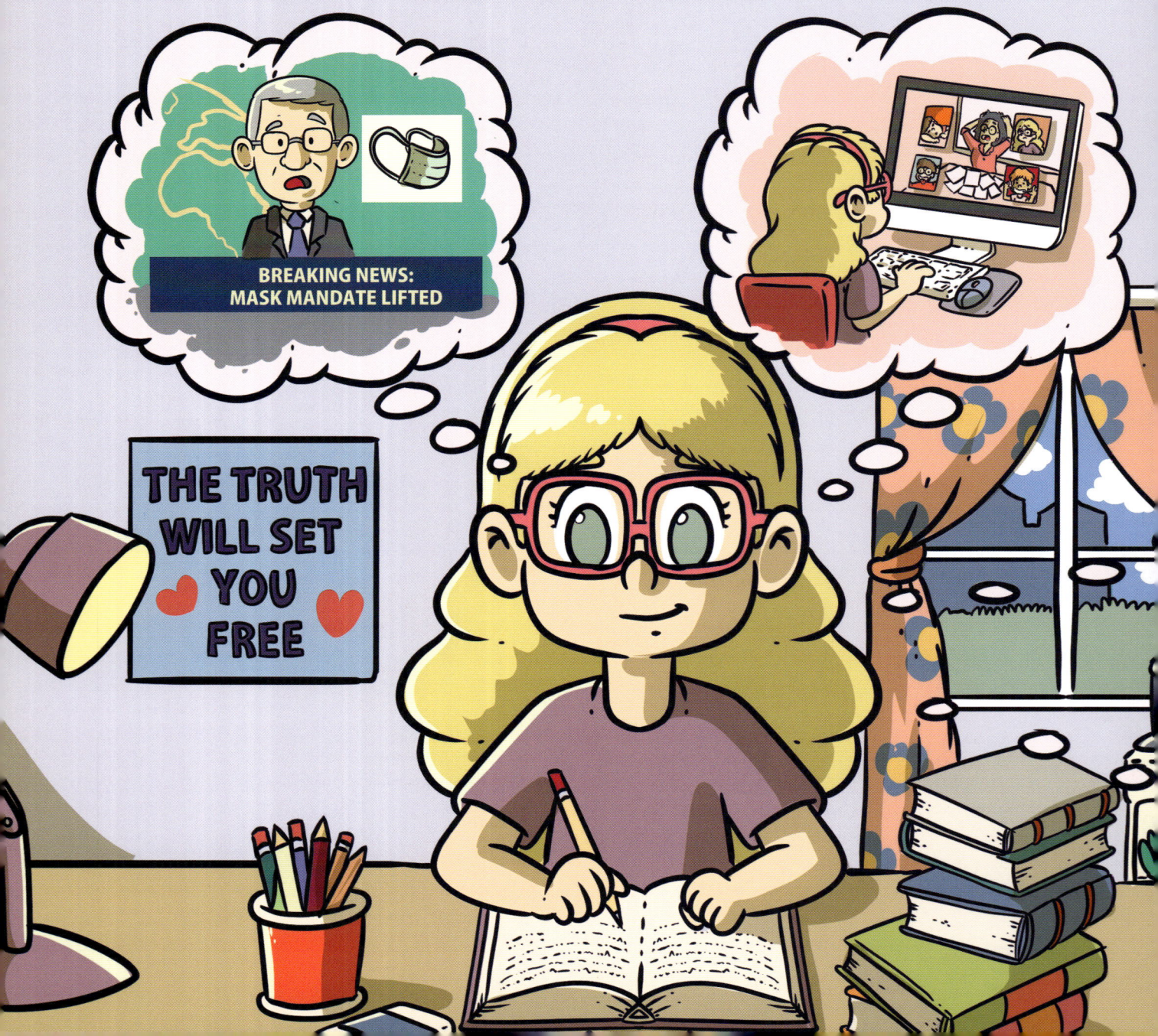

Critical thinking is an important life skill to understand because there will be times in life when we are told to do something that may not make sense, or might go against our beliefs, or violate our freedoms—times when trusting our gut can guide us toward the truth.

Knowing how to think critically about new information, along with listening to our instincts, will help us make smarter choices and ensure a more successful future!

Let's be critical thinkers!

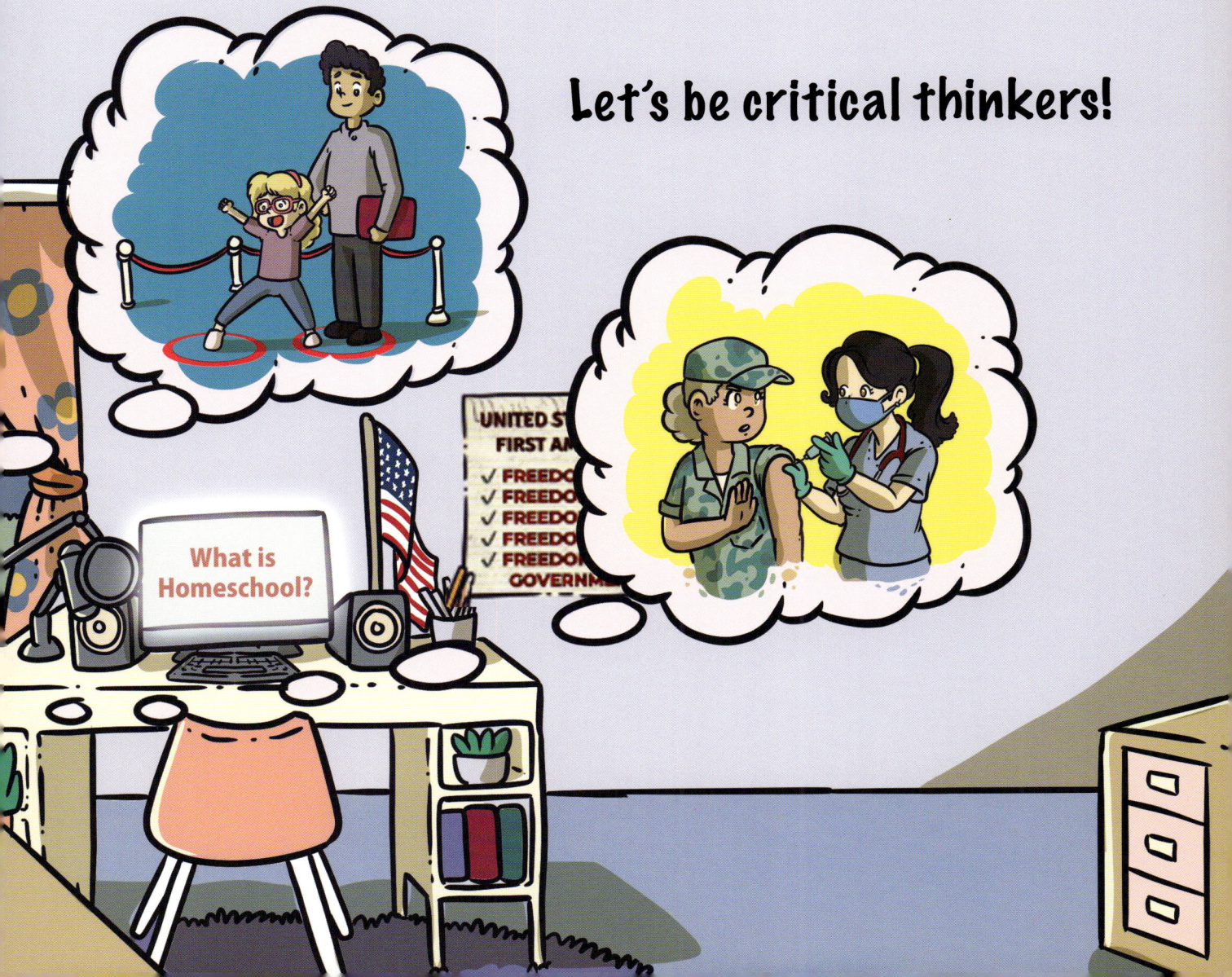

GLOSSARY

<u>Analyze</u>: to separate into parts for close study or examination

<u>Argument</u>: a reason or the reasoning given for or against a matter under discussion

<u>Censorship</u>: when you are purposely prevented from seeing something or saying something

<u>Controversy</u>: a discussion or argument expressing opposing views

<u>Critical thinking</u>: thinking carefully about a subject or idea, without allowing feelings or personal opinions to affect a viewpoint

<u>Emotional response</u>: a reaction to something based on emotions

<u>Evidence</u>: facts, information, or documents that prove something to be true

<u>Fact-check</u>: investigating information to verify facts

<u>Fake news</u>: news stories that are fabricated and are without verifiable facts or resources

<u>Government</u>: a group of people who have the authority to make decisons and create laws to help keep a country or state safe and organized

<u>Informed consent</u>: the process by which a health-care provider educates the patient about risks, benefits, and alternative treatments

<u>Investigative journalist</u>: a type of journalist who does research looking to discover information of public interest

<u>Lockdowns</u>: an emergency situation in which people are not allowed to freely enter or leave a specific location

<u>Logic</u>: thinking carefully about something to see if it makes sense

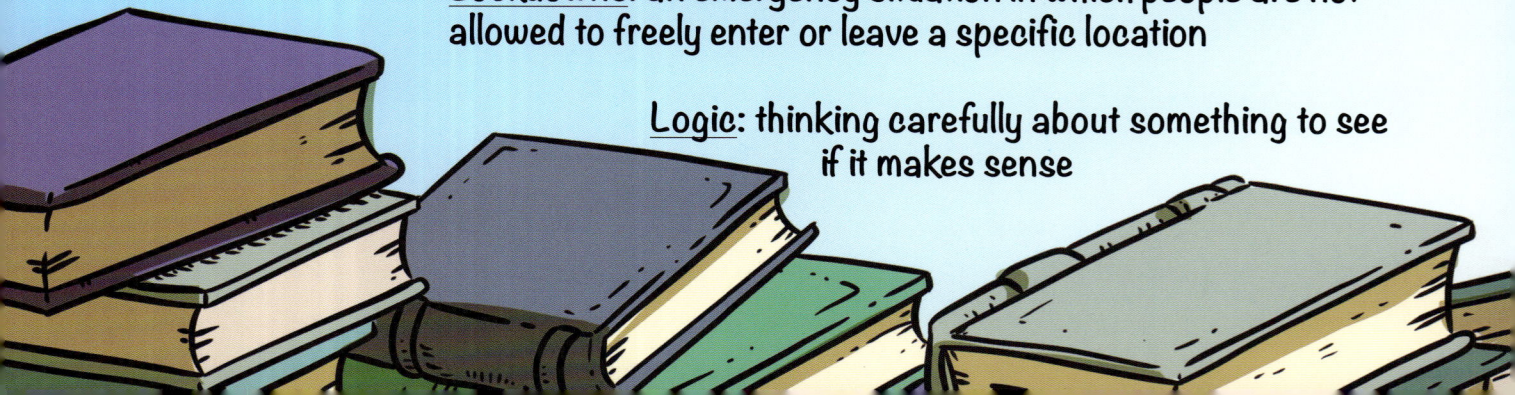

Mandate: an authoritative command or formal order

mRNA technology: technology that uses special molecules called messenger RNA to give the cells in your body specific instructions on how to make proteins

Opinion: a personal thought or belief about something or someone

Pandemic: an outbreak of an infectious disease that spreads among many people over a wide geographical area

Particles: the smallest pieces of matter that make up atoms and parts of atoms

Politician: a person who is elected to help solve problems and make important decisions for states and countries

Propaganda: information, ideas, opinions, or images that often only give one part of an argument and are broadcast, published, or in some other way spread with the intention of influencing people's opinions

Psychologist: a person who specializes in the study of mind and behavior or in the treatment of mental, emotional, or behavioral disorders

Rational response: the use of rational reasoning and understanding when responding

Research: the act of looking for facts and information to learn something new

Surgeon general: someone who has been appointed to oversee public health

Vaccine (CDC definition before 2020): a product that stimulates a person's immune system to produce immunity to a specific disease, protecting the person from that disease

Vaccine (CDC definition after 2020): a preparation that is used to stimulate the body's immune response against diseases

Virus: a tiny germ that can spread and make people and animals sick

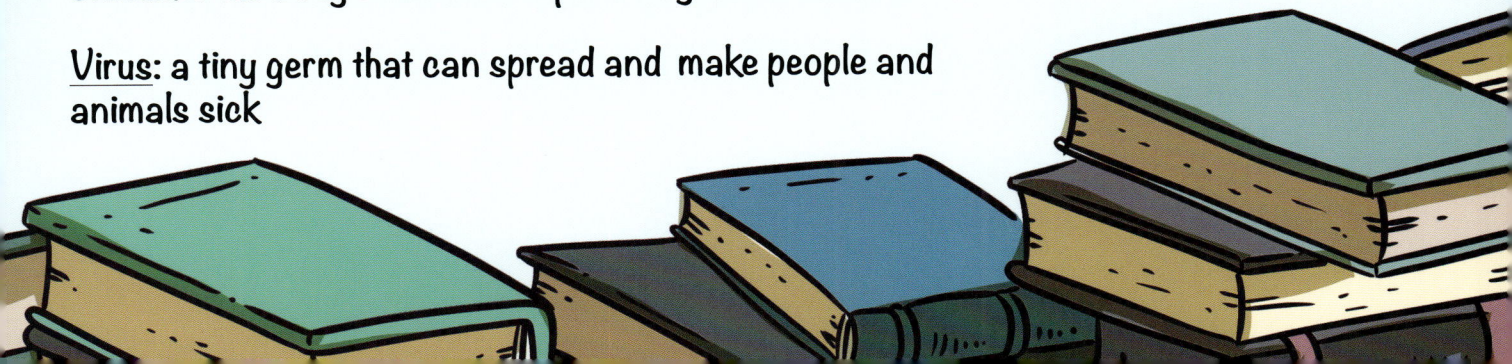

REFERENCES

60 Minutes. "March 2020: Dr. Anthony Fauci Talks with Dr. Jon LaPook about Covid-19," *60 Minutes*, CBS. March 8, 2020. https://www.cbsnews.com/video/march-2020-dr-anthony-fauci-talks-with-dr-jon-lapook-about-covid-19/.

Asadi, S., Wexler, A.S., Cappa, C.D. et al. "Aerosol emission and superemission during human speech increase with voice loudness." *Sci Rep* 9, 2348. 2019. https://doi.org/10.1038/s41598-019-38808-z.

Bazant, M. Z., & Bush, J. W. M. "Beyond six feet: A guideline to limit indoor airborne transmission of COVID-19." medRxiv (Cold Spring Harbor Laboratory). 2020. https://doi.org/10.1101/2020.08.26.20182824.

Central Florida Public Media. Joe Mario Pedersen. "Ladapo's questions on DNA integration with Covid Vax raise experts' eyebrows." January 16, 2024. *Health News Florida.* https://health.wusf.usf.edu/health-news-florida/2024-01-16/ladapos-questions-on-dna-integration-with-covid-vax-raise-experts-eyebrows.

Herby, J., Jonung, L., & Hanke, S. "A Literature Review and Meta-Analysis of the Effects of Lockdowns on COVID-19 Mortality - II." 2023. medRxiv.

Jefferson T, Dooley L, Ferroni E, Al-Ansary LA, van Driel ML, Bawazeer GA, Jones MA, Hoffmann TC, Clark J, Beller EM, Glasziou PP, Conly JM. "Physical interventions to interrupt or reduce the spread of respiratory viruses." Cochrane Database of Systematic Reviews 2023, Issue 1. Art. No.: CD006207. DOI: 10.1002/14651858.CD006207.pub6.

jum934, A. "The impact of the COVID-19 pandemic on children's mental health." *Population Mental Health.* April 22, 2022. https://www.hsph.harvard.edu/population-mental-health/2022/03/07/the-impact-of-the-covid-19-pandemic-on-childrens-mental-health/.

Kluger, J. "How school closures damaged U.S. children's mental health." *Time.* April 29, 2021. https://time.com/5964671/school-closing-children-mental-health-pandemic/.

National Academies of Sciences. "Evidence review of the adverse effects of COVID-19 vaccination and intramuscular vaccine administration." *The National Academies Press.* April 16, 2024. https://doi.org/10.17226/27746.

Singh, S., Roy, D., Sinha, K., Parveen, S., Sharma, G., & Joshi, G. "Impact of COVID-19 and lockdown on mental health of children and adolescents: A narrative review with recommendations." *Psychiatry Research*, 293, 113429. 2020. https://doi.org/10.1016/j.psychres.2020.113429.

"Wenstrup releases statement following Dr. Fauci's two-day testimony." United States House Committee on Oversight and Accountability. January 10, 2024. https://oversight.house.gov/release/wenstrup-releases-statement-follow ing-dr-faucis-two-day-testimony/.

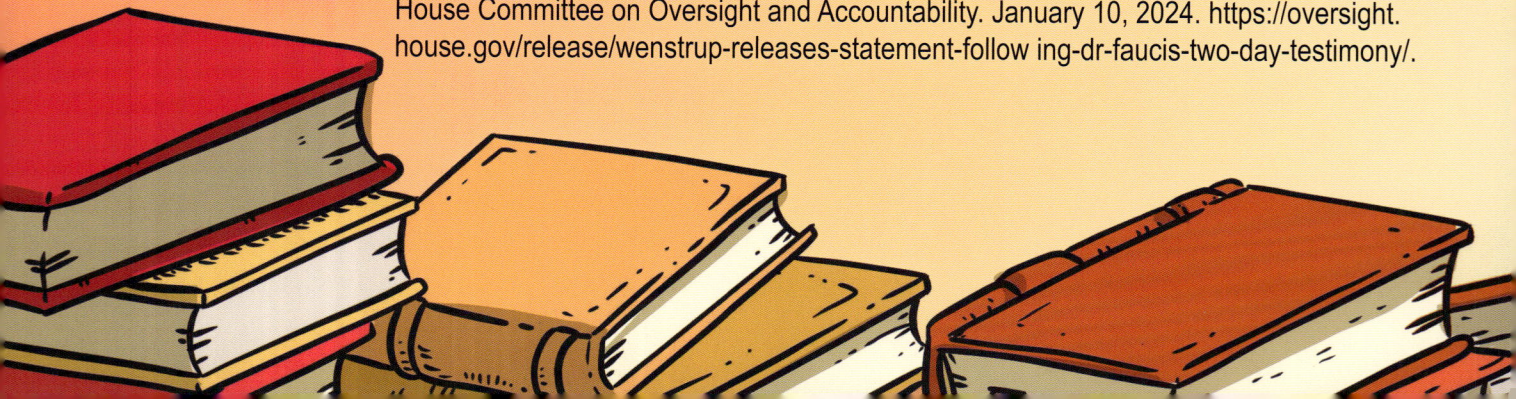

Meet the Author and Illustrator

Dr. Shannon Kroner has a passion for writing children's books that emphasize truth and freedom. She holds a doctorate in clinical psychology, a master's in special education, and a bachelor's in English literature. Dr. Kroner has dedicated much of her career to assisting children with disabilities in a therapeutic setting. She has also taught high school biology and college humanities courses.

As a committed homeschool mom, the executive director of FOR-US, and the author of the award-winning, bestselling children's book, *I'm Unvaccinated and That's OK!*, Dr. Kroner continues to inspire and educate people of all ages.

For more information on Dr. Kroner, , visit drshannonkroner.com or scan the QR code.

AUTHOR

ILLUSTRATOR

Manfred Calderón is a Costa Rican artist, writer, and musician. Fluent in both Spanish and English, Manfred has taught high school art and English classes. He has authored and illustrated a number of his own books. Manfred is also the illustrator of Dr. Kroner's previous book, *I'm Unvaccinated and That's OK!*

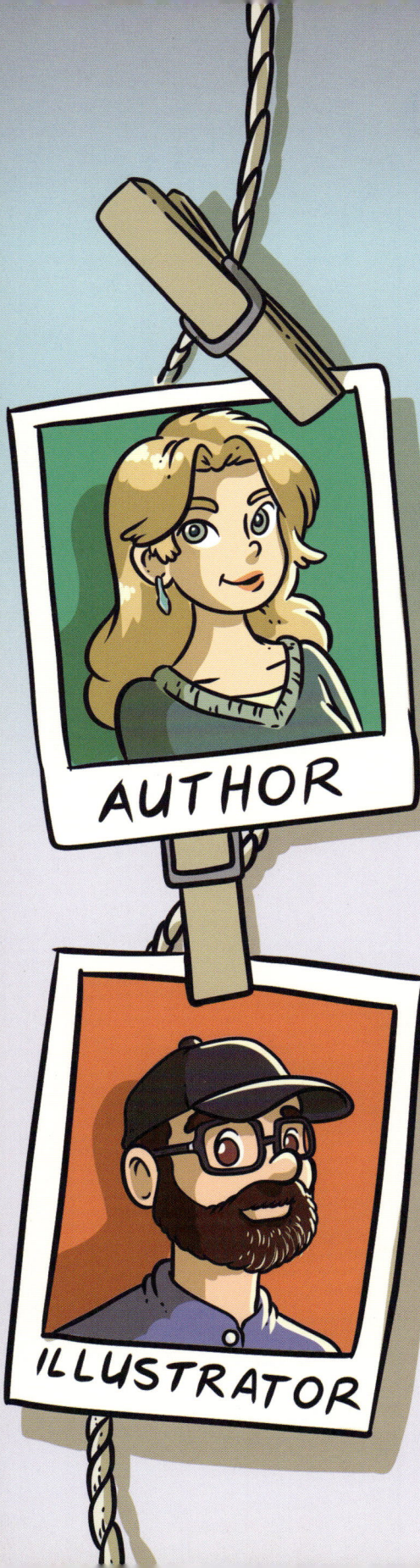

Critical Thinking Activities

1. What are the scientists repeating on page 17 that makes this propaganda?

_____

2. What is the politician saying on page 17 that makes this propaganda?

_____

Can you find any characters from Dr. Kroner's book,
I'm Unvaccinated and That's OK?

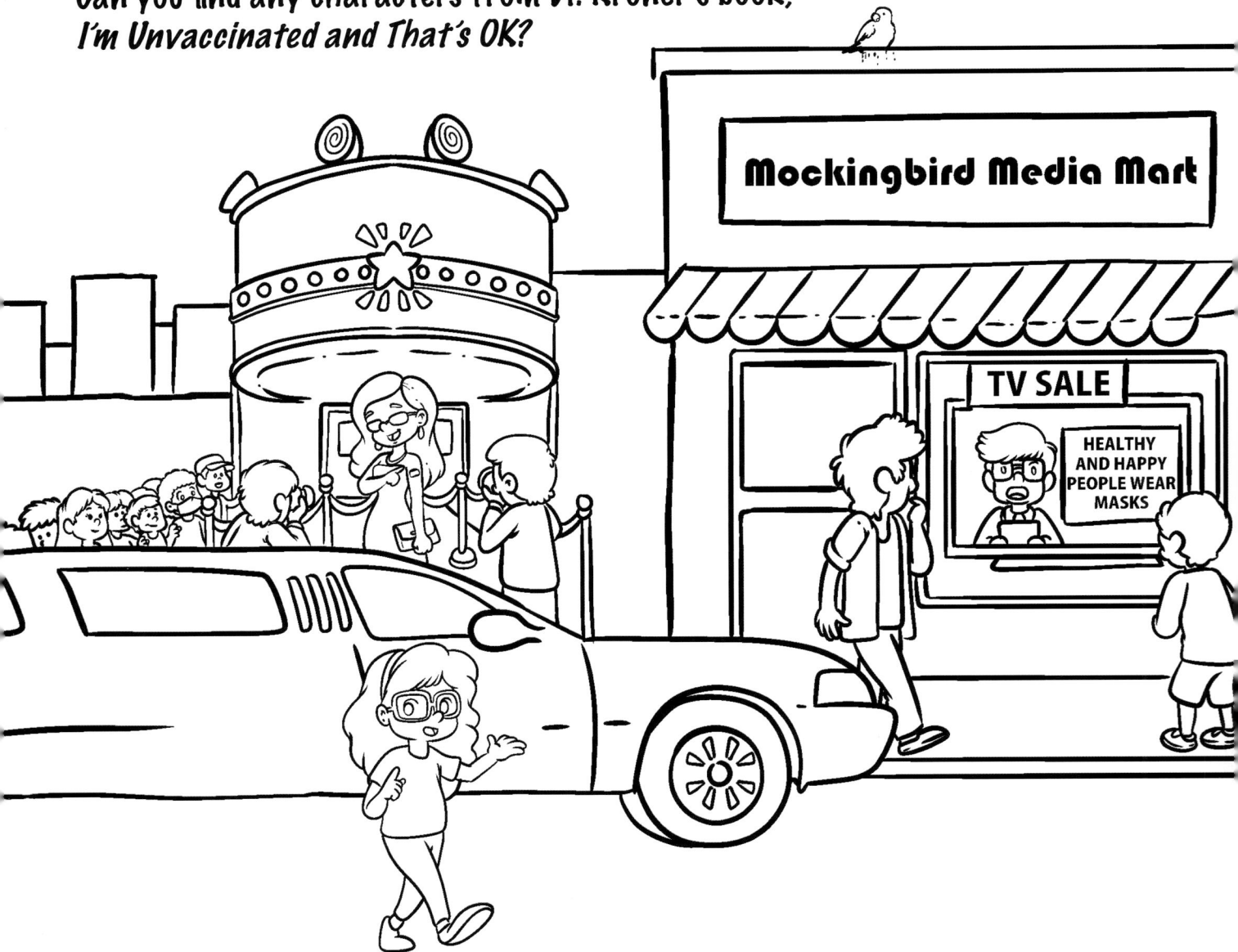

Mockingbird Media Mart

TV SALE

HEALTHY AND HAPPY PEOPLE WEAR MASKS

Color the picture and circle the six examples of people and images spreading propaganda.

1. Actress showing off her vaccination bandage
2. TV in the window
3. Airplane banner
4. Scientists
5. Billboard
6. Politician

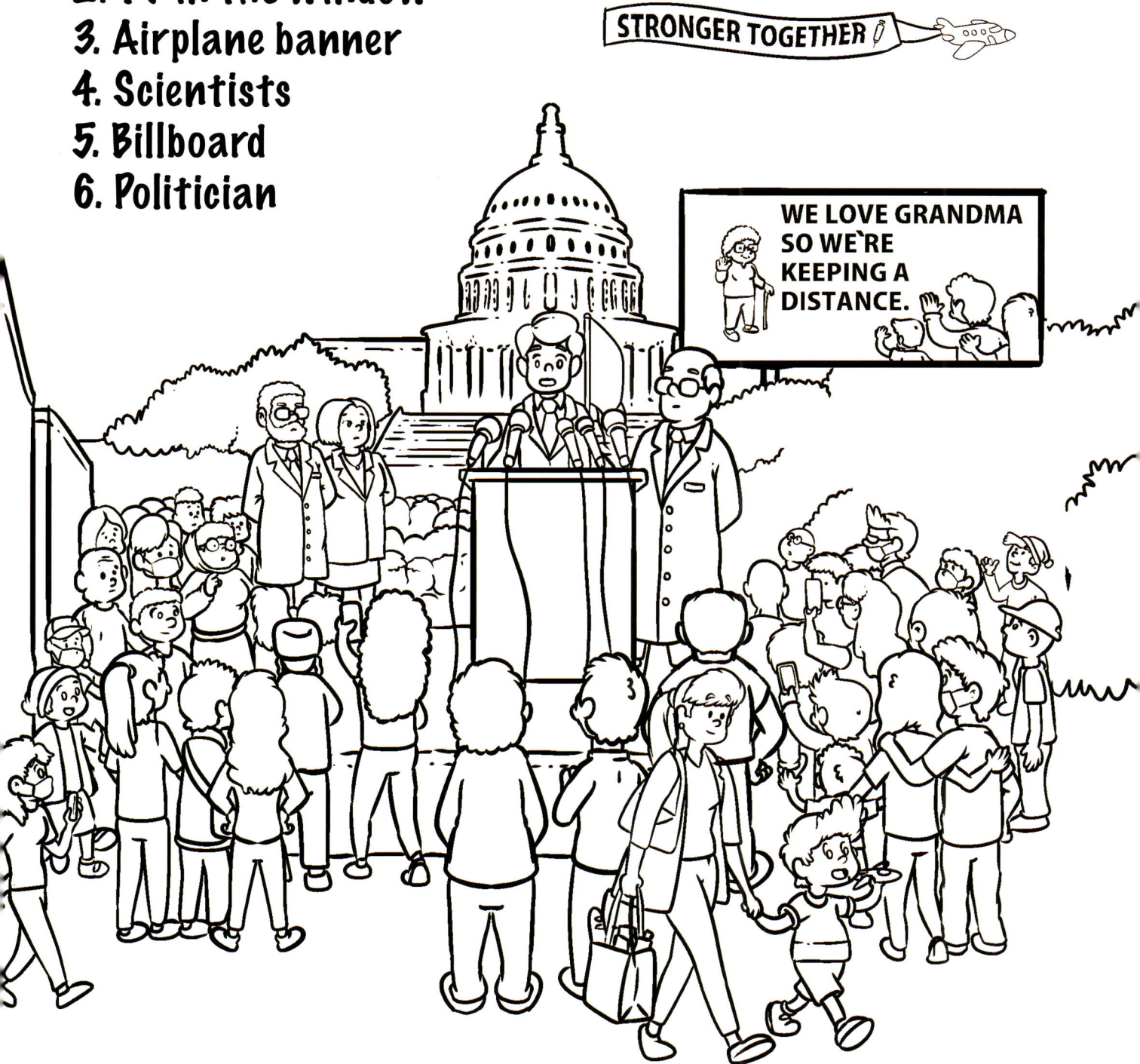

STRONGER TOGETHER

WE LOVE GRANDMA SO WE'RE KEEPING A DISTANCE.

Help Darlene get home safely by avoiding the propaganda.

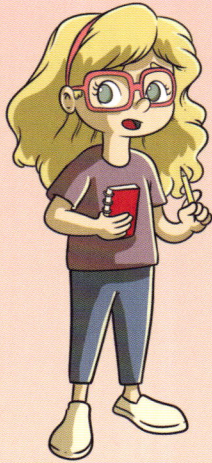

START

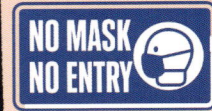

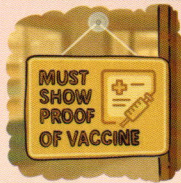

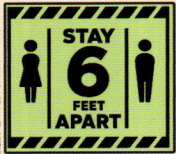

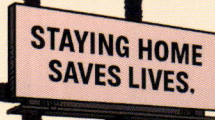

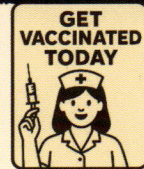

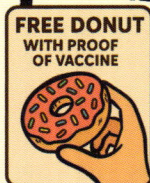

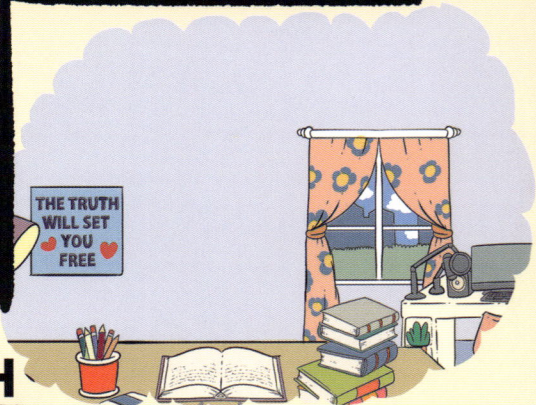

FINISH

While investigating the pandemic, Darlene learned lots of new information using critical thinking skills. Fill in the speech bubbles with what you believe everyone is saying.

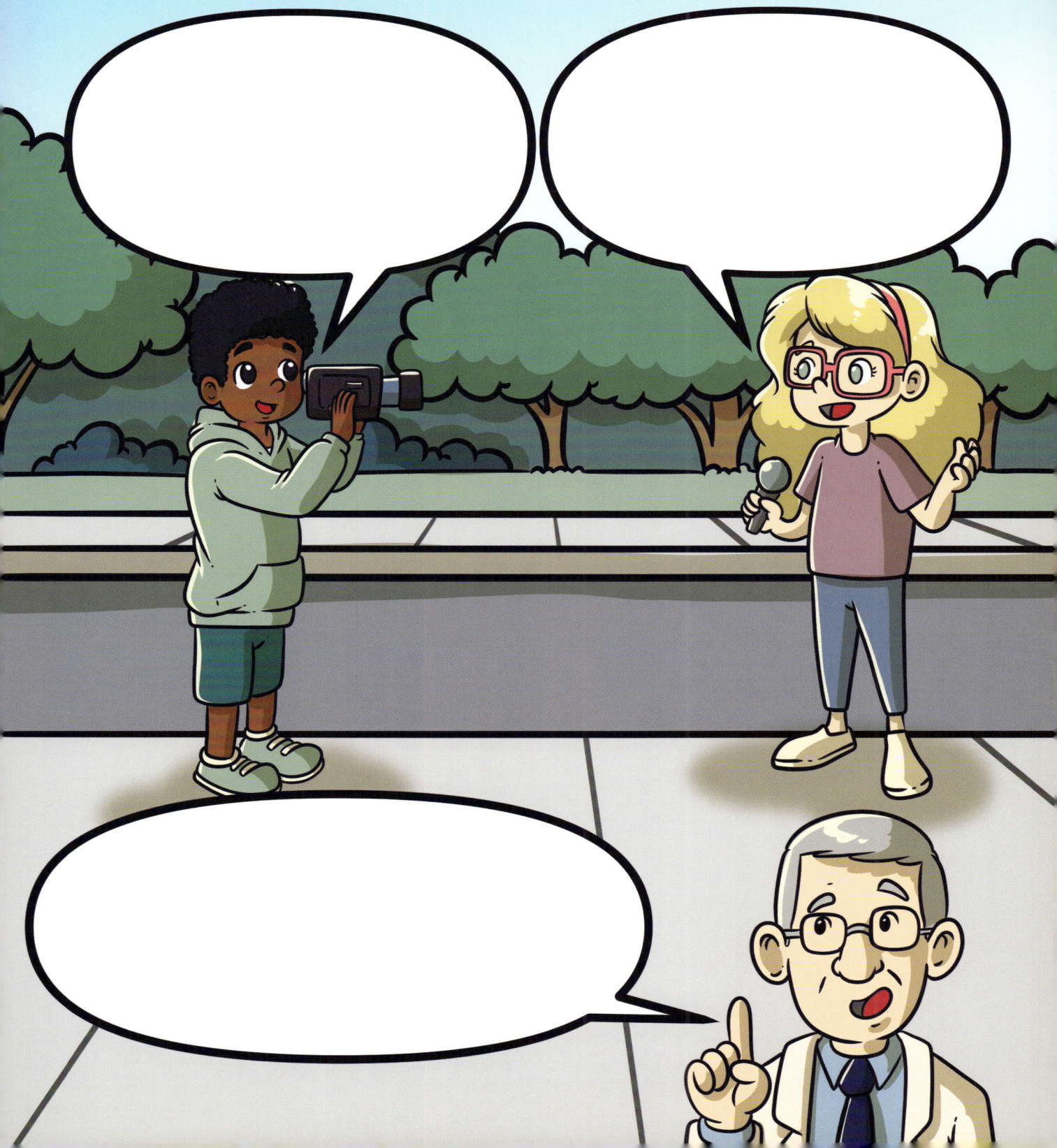

Critical Thinking Exercise

Use this mind map to help investigate your own critical thinking questions.

What do you want to discover?

What is your own opinion about this subject?

Where can you find research related to this question (Websites, books, interviews)?

What does the current research say?

Are there any conflicts of Interest or financial ties that may sway the research?

What did you discover? Do you agree?

More Wise Words from Critical Thinkers

"In an era of information overload, the ability to discern fact from fiction is more critical than ever. Dr. Shannon Kroner's *Let's Be Critical Thinkers* is a vital guide, particularly for young minds navigating complex issues. Through the engaging narrative of Darlene Data, Dr. Kroner skillfully introduces the core principles of critical thinking, empowering readers to question, investigate, and form their own opinions. As a physician with decades of experience, I've witnessed firsthand the importance of pragmatic, evidence-based decision-making. This book champions that approach, encouraging readers to analyze information, identify propaganda, and consider multiple perspectives before drawing conclusions. In a world where narratives are often shaped by agendas, Dr. Kroner equips the next generation with the tools they need to think independently and arrive at the truth. *Let's Be Critical Thinkers* is an essential read for parents and educators seeking to cultivate informed, discerning, and empowered citizens."
—PIERRE KORY, MD, MPH, chief medical officer, Rebuild Medicine, and co-founder Leading Edge Clinic

"Dr. Shannon Kroner's *Let's Be Critical Thinkers* is a sharp hit against the COVID fog of lies—teaching kids to cut through propaganda and challenge the elites with clear-eyed reason. It's a liberty lesson that unmasks the mandate madness, and I'm proud to support this patriot's second book."
—ROGER STONE, political strategist, bestselling author, and presidential campaign advisor

"*Let's Be Critical Thinkers* is a winner—guiding kids to see through mainstream media propaganda with clear eyes and strong hearts. It's a knockout for the next generation, showing them how to hold on to liberty in a world with so much confusion and fake news. I'm proud to back Dr. Kroner's newest book that's bound to be a bestseller."
—TITO ORTIZ, former five-time light heavyweight champion UFC, owner of Tito's Cantina, and motivational speaker

"It's so great that Dr. Shannon Kroner continues to write children's books, giving parents an option for informational books that promote independent thought in a world of conformity and propaganda."
—OWEN SHROYER, *The War Room*, **political talk show host, and journalist**

"Dr. Kroner's *Let's Be Critical Thinkers* is well done and so important. This book provides a helpful tool that teaches both adults and children critical thinking skills in a gentle yet profound way. As we awaken to the deceptive programming all around us, I wish someone had read this book to me as a child. It's a vital guide for kids navigating today's media world, and I'm proud to support my friend's work."
—RICKY SCHRODER, founder of Reel American Heroes, actor, and filmmaker

"*Let's Be Critical Thinkers* is pure gold for parents who value freedom. Dr. Shannon Kroner gives kids the tools to unravel propaganda and rethink pandemic policies—bold, smart, and timely. Sensational and a must for every family's bookshelf!"
—NICK ADAMS, presidential appointee, bestselling author of *The American Boomerang*, **and CEO of Foundation for Liberty and American Greatness**

"Dr. Shannon Kroner has written the essential guide for children to understand the truth and the lies regarding COVID-19. This exploration into critical thinking as applied to masks, lockdowns, social distancing, and vaccination is fun and entertaining while providing vital information and skills to our most vulnerable population. Dr. Kroner's thoughtful book gives children rationality, stability, and calm in the face of the fear, uncertainty, and lies peddled during the pandemic."
—**BRIAN HOOKER, PhD, chief scientific officer of Children's Health Defense**

"In a society where the narratives of a corrupt educational system, the media, and social 'influencers' are revered above one's own observations, ethics, and ability to reason, it is crucial to raise children with the capacity to think critically and sharply question what they are told. Too many kids today are being raised with a dangerous inability to ask the important questions, do their own research, and separate fact from fiction—and Dr. Kroner's powerful book guides them through this essential process. Since the modern education system actively discourages intellectual curiosity and rewards compliance over competence, we must teach our children to think for themselves if humanity is to have a future."
—**BRIANNA LADAPO, MLA, CHC, DAIS, author of *Emerging from Darkness: A Spiritual Memoir and Guide Back to the Light*, naturopath, and healer**

"Dr. Shannon Kroner is at it again, delivering another essential lesson for our children. In a world shaped by relentless propaganda, it's more important than ever to equip the next generation with critical thinking skills. I can't wait for my son to read this—learning to question, analyze, and think independently is invaluable."
—**JESSICA SUTTA, former member of PCD, creative director for React19, and vaccine injury advocate**

"As a child, my parents taught me to be a critical thinker. As a parent, I taught my children to be critical thinkers. As an Air Force officer, the military required me to be a critical thinker. *Let's be Critical Thinkers* creatively captures this conundrum where these expectations for critical thought were turned upside down when it comes to medical choice protected by federal law during the COVID-era. Despite this historic example of disappointing abandonment of these characteristics by institutional forces, Dr. Kroner's brilliant book reminds children that you must have the courage and perseverance to always think critically, act honorably, and never compromise your intellectual integrity."
—**THOMAS L. "BUZZ" REMPFER, colonel, US Air Force (retired)**

"I wish we lived in a world where kids don't have to be equipped to battle propaganda posing as science, but Covid taught us how badly we need the lessons in this book. In fact, far too many adults still need to come to terms with their failure to be critical thinkers. We have work to do, and this brave book plans to get it done."
—**STEVE DEACE, *The Blaze*, TV host, and bestselling author**

"As a military physician, I've witnessed the pressures service members face and the critical need for informed consent. Dr. Shannon Kroner's *Let's Be Critical Thinkers* is a must-read for children and parents. This engaging book empowers kids to question, reason, and understand their medical choices, fostering critical thinking and protecting God-given rights."
—**DR. THERESA M. LONG, MD, MPH, FS**